SpringerBriefs in Public Health

SpringerBriefs in Child Health

Series Editor

Angelo P. Giardino, Salt Lake City, UT, USA

SpringerBriefs in Public Health present concise summaries of cutting-edge research and practical applications from across the entire field of public health, with contributions from medicine, bioethics, health economics, public policy, biostatistics, and sociology.

The focus of the series is to highlight current topics in public health of interest to a global audience, including health care policy; social determinants of health; health issues in developing countries; new research methods; chronic and infectious disease epidemics; and innovative health interventions.

Featuring compact volumes of 50 to 125 pages, the series covers a range of content from professional to academic. Possible volumes in the series may consist of timely reports of state-of-the art analytical techniques, reports from the field, snapshots of hot and/or emerging topics, elaborated theses, literature reviews, and in-depth case studies. Both solicited and unsolicited manuscripts are considered for publication in this series.

Briefs are published as part of Springer's eBook collection, with millions of users worldwide. In addition, Briefs are available for individual print and electronic purchase.

Briefs are characterized by fast, global electronic dissemination, standard publishing contracts, easy-to-use manuscript preparation and formatting guidelines, and expedited production schedules. We aim for publication 8–12 weeks after acceptance.

More information about this series at http://www.springer.com/series/10138

Tanya S. Hinds • Angelo P. Giardino

Child Sexual Abuse

Current Evidence, Clinical Practice, and Policy Directions

With Contributions by Paige A. Culotta,
Marcella M. Donaruma-Kwoh, and Reena Isaac

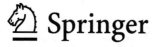 Springer

Tanya S. Hinds
Child & Adolescent Protection Center
Children's National Hospital
Washington, DC, USA

Angelo P. Giardino
Department of Pediatrics
University of Utah School of Medicine
Salt Lake City, UT, USA

ISSN 2625-2872 ISSN 2625-2880 (electronic)
SpringerBriefs in Child Health
ISSN 2192-3698 ISSN 2192-3701 (electronic)
SpringerBriefs in Public Health
ISBN 978-3-030-52548-4 ISBN 978-3-030-52549-1 (eBook)
https://doi.org/10.1007/978-3-030-52549-1

This Springer imprint is published by the registered company Springer Nature Switzerland AG
The registered company address is: Gewerbestrasse 11, 6330 Cham, Switzerland

This monograph is dedicated to our colleague Christopher S. Greeley, MD, MS, FAAP, who is a Professor of Pediatrics at Baylor College of Medicine where he serves as the Section Chief for Public Health Pediatrics and Director of Child Abuse Services at Texas Children's Hospital in Houston, TX. Dr. Greeley provides formidable leadership to the field of Child Abuse Pediatrics and has served as the President of the Helfer Society between 2014 and 2019. He also served as Board Chair for Prevent Child Abuse America between 2009 and 2013. A consummate academic physician, Chris is always willing to offer mentorship to trainees and junior colleagues, focused on the quality of the evidence being used to make clinical decisions, and consistently articulate about the urgency to provide care to all children in our midst regardless of their circumstance.

Preface

In 1981, the U.S. Select Panel for the Promotion of Child Health observed that children are about one-third of our population but all or essentially 100% of our future (1981). By any standard of child health and wellness, that future should be free of child maltreatment, which includes being free from the adversity of child sexual abuse (CSA). The Centers for Disease Control and Prevention defines CSA broadly as the involvement of a child (person less than 18 years old) in sexual activity that they do not fully comprehend, are not developmentally prepared for, and to which they cannot give informed consent (CDC, 2019). The reported incidence of CSA varies by definition and data source, but between at least 58,114 and 135,300 children are sexually abused each year in the United States (USDHHS, 2019; Sedlak et al., 2010). The estimates of prevalence also vary, but approximately 10% of US adults—14% of females and 6% of males—report having been sexually abused prior to reaching 18 years of age (Murray, Nguyen, & Cohen 2014; Finkelhor, Turner, Shattuck, & Hamby, 2015). The impact of being sexually abused includes serious health and wellness consequences such as anxiety, depression, and post-traumatic stress disorder. Healthcare providers have a significant role to play along with the professional disciplines involved with child protection: law enforcement, the courts, and a host of child advocates working in the community and policy realms. This monograph seeks to strike a balance between the conceptual and the practical as well as a balance between the skills needed for individual clinical work with a specific patient and the more broadly based approach necessary for population-level public health policy initiatives.

In order to reach that balance, Chapter 1 provides an overview of the scope of the problem in terms of incidence and prevalence, as well as the variety of risk factors that underlie the issue of CSA. Chapter 2 provides a clinical primer around what a healthcare evaluation would entail for a child suspected of having been sexually abused. Chapter 3 addresses a number of related issues such as delayed disclosure by children who are sexually abused, the accuracy of the details provided by the child during the healthcare interview, the risk of CSA for children with disabilities, the underlying issues surrounding the backlash against child protection professionals investigating CSA cases, and finally, the risk of the internet related to online solicitation of children. Chapter 4 confronts the challenges that health professionals face as they conduct evaluations of children suspected of having been sexually abused. Finally, Chapter 5 talks about policy goals related to CSA prevention—essentially stopping CSA prior to it happening. This chapter also discusses the sea change occurring now in the CSA prevention arena where child-focused personal safety programs are being supplemented with adult-focused training and education that seek to shift the burden of CSA prevention from the potential child victim to the responsible adults who are monitoring and supervising the child's environment. In the end, all children should have futures that embody what the CDC describes as safe, stable, nurturing environments. That noble goal requires everyone, those in the public, professionals who work with children, and the children's caregivers, to continue to take the reality of CSA risk seriously and worthy of attention and effort to prevent. In pediatrics, when working with children, we are trained to be aware that one never knows when they are creating a memory in the experience and mind of a child with whom they are interacting. It is our sincere desire that those who read this monograph and who are called upon to help evaluate a child suspected of having been sexually abused will be better equipped to create a memory of care and concern for that child. In order for that to occur, however, the healthcare professional will need to develop their evaluation skills and will need to practice in a professional and community environment that has resources and policies directed at supporting the child through a difficult process and one that prioritizes their care and well-being. Ultimately, if we can embrace a prevention approach, our hope is that monographs such as this will be less and less necessary as we focus instead on how best to create safe, stable, and nurturing environments that are free from child maltreatment, including CSA.

Washington, DC, USA   Tanya S. Hinds
Salt Lake City, UT, USA   Angelo P. Giardino
March 2020

References

Centers for Disease Control and Prevention, National Center for Injury Prevention and Control, Division of Violence Protection (CDC) (2019). *Preventing child sexual abuse*. Retrieved from www.cdc.gov/violenceprevention/childabuseandneglect/childsexualabuse.html

Finkelhor, D., Turner, H. A., Shattuck, A., & Hamby, S. L. (2015). Prevalence of childhood exposure to violence, crime, and abuse: Results from the national survey of children's exposure to violence. *JAMA Pediatrics, 169*(8), 746–754. https://doi.org/10.1001/jamapediatrics.2015.0676.

Murray, L. K., Nguyen, A., & Cohen, J. A. (2014). Child sexual abuse. *Child and Adolescent Psychiatric Clinics of North America, 23*(2), 321–337. https://doi.org/10.1016/j.chc.2014.01.003.

Sedlak, A. J., Mettenburg, J., Basena, M., Petta, I., McPherson, K., Greene, A., & Li, S. (2010). *Fourth National Incidence Study of child abuse and neglect (NIS–4): Report to congress, executive summary*. Washington, DC: U.S. Department of Health and Human Services,

Administration for Children and Families. Retrieved from http://www.acf.hhs.gov/sites/default/files/opre/nis4_report_congress_full_pdf_jan2010.pdf.

U.S. Department of Health & Human Services, Administration for Children and Families, Administration on Children, Youth and Families, Children's Bureau (USDHHS). (2019). *Child Maltreatment*, 2017. Retrieved from https://www.acf.hhs.gov/cb/research-data-technology/statistics-research/child-maltreatment.

United States Select Panel for the Promotion of Child Health & United States Office of the Assistant Secretary for Health. (1981). *Better health for our children: a national strategy: the report of the Select Panel for the Promotion of Child Health to the United States Congress and the Secretary of Health and Human Services*. Washington, DC: U.S. Dept. of Health and Human Services, Public Health Service, Office of the Assistant Secretary for Health and Surgeon General.

Acknowledgments

The monograph in the SpringerBriefs in Child Health series takes a great deal of effort to produce. It takes a team of academic editors, contributors, and an editorial publishing team to construct the scholarly work that is contained in these pages. The authors express gratitude to Brandy Harman who serves as an academic editor and writing coach in the Department of Pediatrics at the University of Utah in Salt Lake City. Brandy has impeccable writing skills and has a knack for tracking down academic resources that enhance the text as well as for formatting text to make it have an impact on the reader. In addition, we would like to thank Janet Kim, MPH, Senior Editor, Public Health, Springer, our managing editor who provides us with constant encouragement to produce the highest quality publications around a wide range of issues related to child health. A monograph does not come together without an editor like Janet who helps the authors stay focused on the end goal, namely an informative text that is readable and engaging and based in a critical review and synthesis of the available academic literature.

Contents

About the Authors

Tanya S. Hinds, MD, MS, FAAP is an Associate Professor of Pediatrics at the George Washington University School of Medicine and Health Sciences in Washington, DC, and a board-certified Child Abuse Pediatrician. She is an Attending Child Abuse Pediatrician at the Child and Adolescent Protection Center at Children's National Hospital in Washington, DC. In addition to patient care, Dr. Hinds serves as the course director of a Child Abuse Pediatrics elective for medical students. Dr. Hinds is an active participant in the District of Columbia's Multidisciplinary Team on Child Abuse. She is also a member of several national organizations including the American Academy of Pediatrics' Section on Child Abuse and Neglect, the American Professional Society on the Abuse of Children, and the Ray E. Helfer Society. Dr. Hinds is part of several child maltreatment research and education efforts at Children's National Hospital, lectures locally and nationally, and testifies in child abuse cases in the District of Columbia, Maryland, and Virginia.

Angelo P. Giardino, MD, PhD, MPH is the Wilma T. Gibson Presidential Professor and Chair of the Department of Pediatrics at the University of Utah's School of Medicine and Chief Medical Officer at Intermountain Primary Children's Hospital in Salt Lake City, Utah. He received his medical degree and doctorate in education from the University of Pennsylvania, completed his residency and fellowship training at the Children's Hospital of Philadelphia (CHOP), earned a Master's in Public Health from the University of Massachusetts, a Master's in Theology from the Catholic Distance University, and a Master's in Public Affairs from the University of Texas-Rio Grande Valley. He holds subspecialty certifications in Pediatrics and Child Abuse Pediatrics from the American Board of Pediatrics. He is also a Certified Physician Executive (CPE) within the American Association for Physician Leadership. He completed the Patient Safety Certificate Program from the Quality Colloquium, is certified in medical quality (CMQ) as designated by the American Board of Medical Quality, and is a Distinguished Fellow of the American College of Medical Quality. Dr. Giardino is a member of the American Academy of Pediatrics Committee on Child Health Finance. He is a recipient of the Fulbright & Jaworski Faculty Excellence Award at Baylor College of Medicine and the 2013 Health Care

Advocacy Award from Doctors for Change in Houston, TX. His academic accomplishments include published articles, chapters, and textbooks on child abuse and neglect, contributions to several national curricula on the evaluation of child maltreatment, and presentations on a variety of pediatric topics at both national and regional conferences. He is a member of several national and regional boards, including Prevent Child Abuse America, Mobilizing Action for Resilient Communities, the U.S. Center for SafeSport, and the National Advisory Council of the Conference of Major Superiors of Men (CMSM) for the U.S. Catholic Church, where he provides advice on how to best protect children from sexual abuse. He is also coeditor of the Children at Risk Journal of Applied Research on Children: Informing Policy for Children at Risk and the Journal of Family Strengths. Previously, Dr. Giardino served for 12 years on the National Review Board for the U.S. Conference of Catholic Bishops, where he chaired the Research Subcommittee, was elected Vice-Chair, and introduced the concept of high reliability as a quality improvement approach to work towards the response, and ultimately the prevention, of child sexual abuse in the church environment. He currently serves on the local review board for the Diocese of Salt Lake City, Utah.

Contributors

Paige A. Culotta, MD is a board-certified pediatrician currently working as a Child Abuse Pediatrician at the Audrey Hepburn CARE Center with Children's Hospital of New Orleans. Dr. Culotta received an undergraduate degree in biology from Louisiana State University in Baton Rouge and went on to complete medical training at the Louisiana State University Health Sciences Center in New Orleans. She completed her pediatrics residency and child abuse fellowship with Baylor College of Medicine at Texas Children's Hospital in Houston. Dr. Culotta has a special interest in teaching and has given numerous lectures in the community as well as to medical students, residents, and staff physicians to promote knowledge and prevention of child abuse. She has an interest in research on medical child abuse with a focus on improved screening and prevention.

Marcella M. Donaruma-Kwoh, MD, FAAP is an Associate Professor of Pediatrics at Baylor College of Medicine in Houston, Texas. After graduating from Texas A&M University, Dr. Donaruma completed medical school at Baylor College of Medicine. She pursued her internship and residency in Pediatrics at St. Louis Children's Hospital in St. Louis, Missouri. She enjoyed serving for a year as one of the Pediatrics program's chief residents and then concluded her training with a fellowship in a new subspecialty that, at that time, was known as Child Protection and Forensic Pediatrics. This subspecialty was christened Child Abuse Pediatrics in 2009 with the seating of the first board certification exam. Dr. Donaruma is board-certified in Pediatrics and Child Abuse Pediatrics. She has been a member of the Texas Children's Hospital Child Protection Team since 2006.

Reena Isaac, MD is an Assistant Professor of Pediatrics at Baylor College of Medicine and a physician on the Child Abuse Pediatrics Team within the Section of Public Health Pediatrics at Texas Children's Hospital. Dr. Isaac completed her pediatrics training at Albert Einstein College of Medicine/Jacobi Medical Center in New York City, and forensic pediatric training at Brown Medical Center in Providence, Rhode Island. Dr. Isaac has conducted numerous medical investigations of suspected medical child abuse cases and has testified as an expert witness in both family and criminal court regarding such cases.

Chapter 1
Incidence and Prevalence of Child Sexual Abuse

1.1 Definition

Child sexual abuse (CSA), as defined by the World Health Organization (WHO), is "the involvement of a child in sexual activity that he or she does not fully comprehend, is unable to give informed consent to, or for which the child is not developmentally prepared, or else that violates the laws or social taboos of society" (WHO, 2006).

1.2 Scope of the Problem

Incidence, prevalence, and recurrence of child sexual victimization vary depending on the definition of sexual victimization, population being studied, and source of data. In the United States, the National Child Abuse and Neglect Data System (NCANDS) is a federally sponsored passive surveillance effort that compiles data annually on incidence of childhood maltreatment, including sexual victimization, from Child Protective Services (CPS) in the 50 states, the District of Columbia, and Puerto Rico (HHS, 2019). NCANDS defines child sexual abuse as involvement of a child less than 18 years in sexual activity to provide gratification or financial benefit to the perpetrator, including contact for sexual purposes, molestation, statutory rape, prostitution, pornography exposure, incest, or other sexually exploitive activities (HHS, 2019). Childhood sexual victimization represents 8.6% of "screened in" reports to CPS (HHS, 2019) (see Fig. 1.1). In fiscal year 2017, approximately 58,114 children across the United States were subject to CPS investigation or alternative CPS response because of suspected sexual abuse (HHS, 2019). NCANDS underreports the incidence of maltreatment because it only compiles data known to CPS. CPS data in turn only reflects offenses committed by someone acting in a caregiving capacity such as a parent or other caregiver.

© The Author(s) 2020
T. S. Hinds, A. P. Giardino, *Child Sexual Abuse*, SpringerBriefs in Public Health, https://doi.org/10.1007/978-3-030-52549-1_1

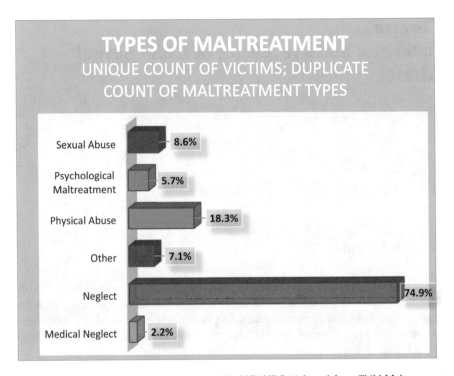

Fig. 1.1 Types of child maltreatment reported by NCANDS (Adapted from Child Maltreatment 2017 by U.S. Department of Health & Human Services Children's Bureau, 2019, Washington, DC)

Over the past two decades, looking at the cases reported to child protective services, Dr. David Finkelhor and colleagues at the University of New Hampshire Crimes Against Children Research Center have studied the trends that emerge from comparing the annual NCANDS reports of substantiated cases (i.e., those children determined to have been maltreated after the case is investigated) (Finkelhor, Saito, & Jones, 2020). Figure 1.2 displays the trend lines from the publicly reported data spanning 1990–2018. Clearly, the graph demonstrates that there is a decreasing trend of substantiated cases of child maltreatment in the United States between 1990 and 2018. Specifically, substantiated cases of sexual abuse have declined by 62%, physical abuse has declined by 53%, and neglect has declined by 11% (Finkelhor et al., 2020).

A great deal of discussion has occurred as to what might be likely causes for this double-digit decline in substantiated cases. Figure 1.3 graphically represents some of the possible contributing factors.

Different from NCANDS' methodology of counting only reported child maltreatment cases, the National Incidence Study of Child Abuse and Neglect (NIS) is an active surveillance effort by the U.S. Department of Health & Human Services that occurs every decade (Sedlak et al., 2010). The NIS compiles CPS data and data from "sentinel" agencies that have regular contact with children, including public

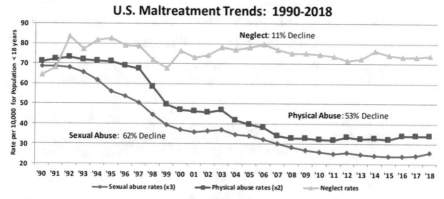

U.S. Maltreatment Trends: 1990-2018

Note: Trend estimates represent total change from 1992 to 2018. Annual rates for physical abuse and sexual abuse have been multiplied by 2 and 3 respectively in Figure 1 so that trend comparisons can be highlighted.

Fig. 1.2 Trends in substantiated child maltreatment cases (Reprinted from *Updated Trends in Child Maltreatment, 2018* by D. Finkelhor et al. 2020, Crimes against Children Research Center, Durham, NC)

schools, medical facilities, and law enforcement agencies across a nationally representative sample of 122 US counties. Compilation of data from these sources thus captures cases that were either "screened out" by CPS or not reported to CPS in addition to "screened in" CPS data. NIS defines child sexual abuse as involvement of a child up to 18 years of age in intrusive sexual contact, molestation with genital contact, attempted or threatened physical contact, or involvement in prostitution, pornography, voyeurism, and/or failure to supervise a child's voluntary sexual activity. NIS data is collected based on two standards: Harm and Endangerment. The Harm Standard refers to an act or an omission resulting in demonstrable harm or injury. For maltreatment to be counted under the Harm Standard, the perpetrator must be a parent, parent substitute, or an adult caretaker. The Endangerment Standard refers to (1) children who meet the Harm Standard, (2) those not yet harmed but thought to be endangered, and (3) cases where a CPS investigation substantiated or indicated a child's maltreatment in spite of lack of demonstrable harm. The Endangerment Standard for sexual abuse enlarges the set of allowable perpetrators by also counting cases in which children were abused by teenage caretakers. Figure 1.4 depicts the NIS data gathering and analysis methodologies.

The most recent study, NIS-4, was published in 2010 and reported on 2005–2006 data (Sedlak et al., 2010). NIS-4 estimated the number of children who experienced Harm Standard sexual abuse decreased from 217,700 in 1993 to 135,300 in 2005–2006; a 38% decrease. The number of children who experienced Endangerment Standard sexual abuse decreased from 300,200 in 1993 to 180,500 in 2005–2006; a 40% decrease (Sedlak et al. 2010) (see Tables 1.1 and 1.2).

It is generally acknowledged that official reports to CPS, law enforcement, and/ or known mandated reporters represent a fraction of childhood sexual victimization. Case ascertainment can also be achieved through screening of parents and/or children about their experiences related to childhood sexual victimization. In a

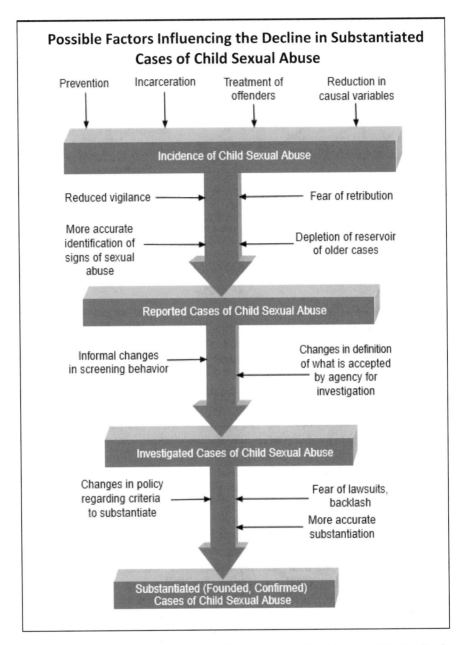

Fig. 1.3 Possible factors in the decline of child sexual abuse (Reprinted from "The Decline in Child Sexual Abuse Cases," by L. Jones and D. Finkehor, Jones & Finkelhor 2001, Juvenile Justice Bulletin, Washington, DC: U.S. Department of Justice)

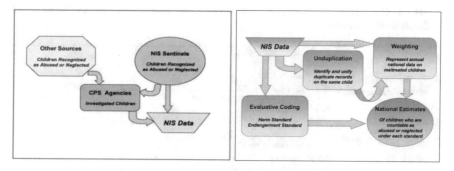

Fig. 1.4 NIS data sources and analysis methodologies (Reprinted from *Fourth National Incidence Study of Child Abuse and Neglect (NIS-4): Report to Congress*, pp. 2–5, 2–6, by A.J. Sedlak et al. 2010, Washington, DC: U.S. Department of Health and Human Services, Administration for Children and Families)

multinational household survey of youth aged 18–24 years, sexual victimization was defined as unwanted touching, attempted sex, coerced sex, and forced sex (Sumner et al. 2015). **The prevalence of sexual victimization before age 18 years exceeded 25% among females in Haiti, Kenya, Swaziland, Tanzania, and Zimbabwe and exceeded 11% among males in Haiti, Kenya, Malawi, and Tanzania** (Sumner et al., 2015). A US-based telephone survey of youth aged 10–17 years and parents of children aged 9 years or younger highlighted the experiences of US children (Finkelhor, Turner, Shattuck, & Hamby, 2015). **Fourteen percent (14%) of American girls and 6% of American boys reported sexual offenses involving contact before age 18 years; completed rape occurred in 4.5% of girls and 0.2% of boys prior to age 18 years** (Finkelhor et al., 2015).

Increasingly, child advocates are becoming more aware of commercial sexual exploitation (CSE), a form of human trafficking, which includes the recruiting, enticing, harboring, transporting, providing, obtaining, and/or maintaining a child for the purpose of sexual exploitation, including prostitution, exchange of sexual acts for something of value, pornography, performance at sexual venues, and/or early marriage (IOM & NRC, 2013). Children are subjected to sex trafficking in a range of venues including red light districts, tourist destinations, vehicles, private homes, religious pilgrimage centers, and mining camps (U.S. Department of State, 2016). International statistics on numbers of children involved in CSE are difficult to determine. Experts estimate millions of women and children are victims of sex trafficking in India alone (U.S. Department of State, 2016).

Among a nationally representative sample of 13,294 US-based seventh to twelfth graders, 3.5% admit to exchanging sex for money or drugs; two-thirds of these teens were male (Edwards, Iritani, & Hallfors, 2006). **Girls in the United States, Canada, and Mexico are typically between 12 and 14 years and boys 11–13 years when they first become victims of CSE** (Estes & Weiner, 2002). **North American youth at increased risk for commercial sex trafficking include female gang**

Table 1.1 Comparison of the national incidence of Harm Standard maltreatment in the NIS-4 with earlier NIS estimates

Harm Standard Maltreatment Category	NIS–4 Estimates 2005–2006		Comparisons With Earlier Studies					
			NIS–3 Estimates 1993			NIS–2 Estimates 1986		
	Total No. of Children	Rate per 1,000 Children	Total No. of Children	Rate per 1,000 Children		Total No. of Children	Rate per 1,000 Children	
ALL MALTREATMENT	1,256,600	17.1	1,553,800	23.1	m	931,000	14.8	ns
ABUSE:								
ALL ABUSE	553,300	7.5	743,200	11.1	*	507,700	8.1	ns
Physical Abuse	323,000	4.4	381,700	5.7	m	269,700	4.3	ns
Sexual Abuse	135,300	1.8	217,700	3.2	*	119,200	1.9	ns
Emotional Abuse	148,500	2.0	204,500	3.0	m	155,200	2.5	ns
NEGLECT:								
ALL NEGLECT	771,700	10.5	879,000	13.1	ns	474,800	7.5	m
Physical Neglect	295,300	4.0	338,900	5.0	ns	167,800	2.7	m
Emotional Neglect	193,400	2.6	212,800	3.2	ns	49,200	0.8	*
Educational Neglect[†]	360,500	4.9	397,300	5.9	ns	284,800	4.5	ns

*	The difference between this and the NIS–4 incidence rate is significant at p≤.05.
m	The difference between this and the NIS–4 incidence rate is statistically marginal (i.e., .10>p>.05).
ns	The difference between this and the NIS–4 incidence rate is neither significant nor marginal (p>.10).
†	Educational neglect is identical under the Harm and Endangerment Standards. It is included in both tables because it is in the summary categories in both standards: All Neglect and All Maltreatment
Note:	Estimated totals are rounded to the nearest 100.

Reprinted from *Fourth National Incidence Study of Child Abuse and Neglect (NIS-4): Report to Congress*, **p. 3–4, by A.J. Sedlak et al. 2010, Washington, DC: U.S. Department of Health and Human Services, Administration for Children and Families**

members and gay, bisexual, and transgender youth (Estes & Weiner, 2002). **Missing children are also at increased risk for commercial sex trafficking.** In the United States, the National Center for Missing and Exploited Children® (NCMEC) runs a 24-hour hotline that accepts reports related to missing and sexually exploited children. NCMEC estimates that 20% of the 11,800 runaways reported to NCMEC in 2015 were likely CSE victims. NCMEC believes 74% of these likely sex trafficking victims were in the care of social services or foster care when they went missing.

Table 1.2 Comparison of the national incidence of Endangerment Standard maltreatment in the NIS-4 with earlier NIS estimates

Endangerment Standard Maltreatment Category	NIS–4 Estimates 2005–2006		Comparisons With Earlier Studies					
			NIS–3 Estimates 1993			NIS–2 Estimates 1986		
	Total No. of Children	Rate per 1,000 Children	Total No. of Children	Rate per 1,000 Children		Total No. of Children	Rate per 1,000 Children	
ALL MALTREATMENT	2,905,800	39.5	2,815,600	41.9	ns	1,424,400	22.6	*
ABUSE:								
ALL ABUSE	835,000	11.3	1,221,800	18.2	*	590,800	9.4	m
Physical Abuse	476,600	6.5	614,100	9.1	*	311,500	4.9	*
Sexual Abuse	180,500	2.4	300,200	4.5	*	133,600	2.1	ns
Emotional Abuse	302,600	4.1	532,200	7.9	*	188,100	3.0	m
NEGLECT:								
ALL NEGLECT	2,251,600	30.6	1,961,300	29.2	ns	917,200	14.6	*
Physical Neglect	1,192,200	16.2	1,335,100	19.9	ns	507,700	8.1	*
Emotional Neglect	1,173,800	15.9	584,100	8.7	*	203,000	3.2	*
Educational Neglect[†]	360,500	4.9	397,300	5.9	ns	284,800	4.5	ns

*	The difference between this and the NIS–4 incidence rate is significant at p≤.05.
m	The difference between this and the NIS–4 incidence rate is statistically marginal (i.e., .10>p>.05).
ns	The difference between this and the NIS–4 incidence rate is neither significant nor marginal (p>.10).
Note:	Estimated totals are rounded to the nearest 100.
†	Educational neglect is identical under the Harm and Endangerment Standards. It is included in both tables because it is in the summary categories in both standards: All Neglect and All Maltreatment.

Reprinted from *Fourth National Incidence Study of Child Abuse and Neglect (NIS-4): Report to Congress*, **p. 3–15, by A.J. Sedlak et al. 2010, Washington, DC: U.S. Department of Health and Human Services, Administration for Children and Families**

1.3   Child, Caregiver, and Environmental Risk Factors

Juveniles make up the greatest proportion of sexual assault victims reported to law enforcement: one-third (32.8%) of all victims were aged 12–17 years at time of report, and another third (34.1%) were under 12 years (Snyder, 2000). One of every seven victims of sexual violence (14%) reported to law enforcement agencies is under 6 years (Snyder, 2000). American victims of in-person child sexual victimization are overwhelmingly female; numbers for males are much lower, in part because males are less likely to officially report sexual abuse or assault (Snyder, 2000). According to law enforcement data, females have six times the rate of sexual abuse or assault compared with males. The data also suggest the **risk of sexual violence** among juvenile females increases with age, peaking for most forms of sexual abuse or assault at 14 years (Snyder, 2000). Reported cases indicate 4 years is the age at which a male is most likely to be the victim of sexual violence (Snyder, 2000).

Nearly all known perpetrators of contact sexual abuse or assault are male, and only 7% of perpetrators of sexual violence against children 17 years or younger are strangers. Perpetrators of child sexual abuse or assault are usually family members (34.2%) or acquaintances (58.7%) of the child or family (Snyder, 2000). In the United States, a known adult is seven times more likely and a known peer 17 times more likely to perpetrate child sexual assault compared with a stranger (Finkelhor et al., 2015). The single age with the highest proportion of offenders was 14 years; however, adults perpetrate 60% of known sexual assaults against children 12 years and younger (Snyder, 2000). Seventy-seven percent (77%) of sexual assaults of juveniles in the United States occur in their homes. American children under 6 years are most likely to be violated between 9 a.m. and 6 p.m. with peaks at 3 p.m. and around traditional meal times of 8 a.m., noon, and 6 p.m. (Snyder, 2000).

College students, particularly undergraduates, are also at increased risk for sexual violence by an acquaintance compared with a stranger. Eight in 10 college student victims are raped by an acquaintance (Warshaw, 1988). Among US college students at a single urban college, 23% of female college students and 11.6% of males disclosed at least one episode of unwanted sexual contact since beginning college; among these students, 6.7% of women and 2.8% of men disclosed rape (Conley et al., 2017). Transgender, genderqueer, non-conforming (TGQN) and questioning college students have a higher risk of sexual violence compared with non-TGQN students (Westat, 2017). Often, unwanted sexual contact and/or rape since beginning college constituted revictimization of the individual. Among the 22% of college students reporting unwanted sexual contact before college, nearly 4 in 10 reported additional unwanted sexual contact or rape since entering college. Females and males had similar rates of revictimization. Among female college students, a history of unwanted sexual contact before college, alcohol use, and depression appeared to increase the risk for sexual victimization during college (Conley et al. 2017). Only a quarter of sexual assaults of college students is reported to law enforcement or campus officials (Westat, 2017).

At present, known internet-facilitated sexual exploitation of children and teens appears to be a fraction of in-person/contact sexual offenses. However, Internet access and technology has helped facilitate online sexual grooming, sexual harassment, and the commercial sexual exploitation of children around the world. Although CSE of children is a form of sexual abuse, children aged 12–18 years involved in CSE differ from child sexual abuse victims without evidence of CSE. Child victims of CSE have significantly higher rates of prior STIs (53%), physical abuse (44%), history of violence with sex (31%), drug or alcohol use (70%), polysubstance use (50%), history of running away from home (81%), and prior involvement with child protective services (47%) and law enforcement (75%) (Varma, Gillespie, McCracken, & Greenbaum, 2015). Tattoos (48%) and a history of a fracture, significant laceration, or traumatic loss of consciousness (32%) are significantly more frequent among CSE victims compared with children where there is suspicion of sexual assault but no suspicion of CSE ($p < 0.001$). Healthcare providers frequently have contact with these children, but may not detect that children are victims. **More than three in four child victims of CSE in New York report they presented for health care because of illness or injury in the previous 6 months** (Curtis, Terry, Dank, Dombrowski, & Khan, 2008).

Child sexual victimization also has intergenerational consequences. Mothers who were sexually abused in their childhood are at increased risk of their children being sexually abused (Oates, Tebbutt, Swanston, Lynch, & O'Toole, 1998). Thirty-four percent (34%) of mothers of sexually abused children disclose a history of sexual abuse in their own childhoods compared with 12% of mothers whose children are not known to have been sexually abused themselves (Oates et al., 1998).

References

Conley, A. H., Overstreet, C. M., Hawn, S. E., Kendler, K. S., Dick, D. M., & Amstadter, A. B. (2017). Prevalence and predictors of sexual assault among a college sample. *Journal of American College Health, 65*(1), 41–49. https://doi.org/10.1080/07448481.2016.1235578.

Curtis, R., Terry, K., Dank, M., Dombrowski, K., & Khan, B. (2008). *The commercial sexual exploitation of children in New York City: Vol. 1.* Washington, D.C.: U.S. Department of Justice. Retrieved from https://www.ncjrs.gov/pdffiles1/nij/grants/225083.pdf.

Edwards, J. M., Iritani, B. J., & Hallfors, D. D. (2006). Prevalence and correlates of exchanging sex for drugs or money among adolescents in the United States. *Sexually Transmitted Infections, 82*(5), 354–358. https://doi.org/10.1136/sti.2006.020693.

Estes, R., & Weiner, N. (2002). *The commercial sexual exploitation of children in the U. S., Canada and Mexico.* Philadelphia: University of Pennsylvania School of Social Work Center for the Study of Youth Policy.

Finkelhor, D., Saito, K., & Jones, L. (2020). *Updated trends in child maltreatment, 2018.* Durham, NH: Crimes against Children Research Center, Durham.

Finkelhor, D., Turner, H. A., Shattuck, A., & Hamby, S. L. (2015). Prevalence of childhood exposure to violence, crime, and abuse: Results from the national survey of children's exposure to violence. *JAMA Pediatrics, 169*(8), 746–754. https://doi.org/10.1001/jamapediatrics.2015.0676.

Institute of Medicine (IOM), National Research Council (NRC). (2013). *Confronting commercial sexual exploitation and sex trafficking of minors in the United States.* Washington, DC: The National Academies Press. https://doi.org/10.17226/18358.

Jones, L., & Finkelhor, D. (2001). *The decline in sexual abuse cases (Juvenile Justice Bulletin—NCJ184741).* Washington, DC: U.S. Government Printing Office. Retrieved from https://scholars.unh.edu/cgi/viewcontent.cgi?article=1005&context=ccrc.

Oates, R. K., Tebbutt, J., Swanston, H., Lynch, D. L., & O'Toole, B. I. (1998). Prior childhood sexual abuse in mothers of sexually abused children. *Child Abuse & Neglect, 22*(11), 1113–1118. https://doi.org/10.1016/s0145-2134(98)00091-X.

Sedlak, A.J., Mettenburg, J., Basena, M., Petta, I., McPherson, K., Greene, A., & Li, S. (2010) Fourth national incidence study of child abuse and neglect (NIS-4): Report to congress. Washington, DC: U.S. Department of Health and Human Services, Administration for Children and Families. Retrieved from http://www.acf.hhs.gov/sites/default/files/opre/nis4_report_congress_full_pdf_jan2010.pdf

Snyder, H. N. (2000) *Sexual assault of young children as reported to law enforcement: Victim, incident, and offender characteristics* (Report No. NCJ 182990). Bureau of Justice Statistics. Retrieved from http://www.bjs.gov/index.cfm?ty=pbdetail&iid=1147

Sumner, S. A., Mercy, A. A., Saul, J., Motsa-Nzuza, N., Kwesigabo, G., Buluma, R. … Centers for Disease Control and Prevention (CDC) (2015) Prevalence of sexual violence against children and use of social services–Seven countries, 2007-2013. *Morbidity and Mortality Weekly Report, 64*(21), 565–569. Retrieved from http://www.cdc.gov/mmwr/pdf/wk/mm6421.pdf.

U.S. Department of Health & Human Services, Administration for Children and Families, Administration on Children, Youth and Families, Children's Bureau (HHS). (2019). *Child maltreatment* (p. 2017). Washington, DC: HHS. Retrieved from https://www.acf.hhs.gov/cb/research-data-technology/statistics-research/child-maltreatment.

U.S. Department of State, Office of the Under Secretary for Civilian Security, Democracy, and Human Rights. (2016). *Trafficking in persons report*. Retrieved from https://www.state.gov/j/tip/rls/tiprpt/2016/

Varma, S., Gillespie, S., McCracken, C., & Greenbaum, V. J. (2015). Characteristics of child commercial sexual exploitation and sex trafficking victims presenting for medical care in the United States. *Child Abuse & Neglect, 44*, 98–105. https://doi.org/10.1016/j.chiabu.2015.04.004.

Warshaw, R. (1988). *I never called it rape: The Ms* (Report on recognizing, fighting, and surviving date and acquaintance rape). New York: HarperCollins.

Westat. (2017). *Report on the AAU climate survey on sexual assault and sexual misconduct*. Retrieved from https://www.aau.edu/Climate-Survey.aspx?id=16525

World Health Organization (WHO). (2006). *Preventing child maltreatment: A guide to taking action and generating evidence*. Retrieved from http://www.who.int/violence_injury_prevention/publications/violence/child_maltreatment

Chapter 2
Clinical Perspective

2.1 Listening and History Taking

Medical history taking has long been regarded as the most important aspect of diagnosis and treatment. Sir William Osler, MD, who helped found the discipline of internal medicine and was instrumental in developing the system of clinical medical education that continues to be used today, advised, "Listen to your patient, he is telling you the diagnosis." Most diagnoses (approximately 80%) are made by careful history taking (Peterson, Holbrook, Von Hales, Smith, & Staker, 1992). This basic medical tenet holds true in the diagnosis of child sexual victimization (child sexual abuse or assault). Among children evaluated for child sexual abuse or assault, only a minority of anogenital examinations, typically 7% or less, have physical findings at the time of examination (Al-Jilaihawi, Borg, Jamieson, Maguire, & Hodes, 2017; Smith, Raman, Madigan, Waldman & Shouldice, 2018; Gallion, Milam, & Littrell, 2016; Heger, Ticson, Velasquez, & Bernier, 2002b; Berenson et al., 2000). Emphasis must be placed on listening and asking open-ended questions of the child and/or caregiver(s) (see Table 2.1).

Listening and history taking must address several overarching concerns when child sexual victimization is suspected: (1) physical safety and risk of additional harm; (2) mental health care; (3) timing of the medical examination; (4) whether or not biologic fluids need to be collected; and, (5) reporting to Child Protective Services (Jenny & Crawford-Jakubiak, 2013). Historical elements can be obtained from the child, caregiver, and/or another involved professional (Table 2.1). The history (and physical examination) should be conducted in the language preferred by the child and caregiver(s). Listening and history taking should be facilitated by a formally trained interpreter when family and clinician do not share family's preferred language. Family members and investigators are not ideal interpreters for these encounters which have medical and legal ramifications.

Most cases of child sexual victimization come to light because of a child's disclosure. A concerning disclosure may be intentional, inadvertent, incremental, or

© The Author(s) 2020
T. S. Hinds, A. P. Giardino, *Child Sexual Abuse*, SpringerBriefs in Public Health, https://doi.org/10.1007/978-3-030-52549-1_2

Table 2.1 Recommended historical elements in the medical evaluation of suspected child sexual victimization[a,b,c]

History of present injury	What, where, when, who
	Associated pain, bleeding, dysuria, discharge
	Suspected perpetrator(s) risks for sexually transmitted infections
	Suspected perpetrator(s) threats of and/or actual force
	Response to child's disclosure by primary caregiver(s)
Review of systems	Suicidality
	Adverse behavioral changes (e.g., sexualized behavior, enuresis, encopresis, school performance)
	Constitutional changes (e.g., appetite, sleep)
	Current symptoms of an oral or anogenital STI
	Non-genital concerns (e.g., abdominal pain, skin injuries)
Past medical history	Medical and mental health diagnoses
	Episode(s) of maltreatment
	Injuries (including straddle or anogenital injuries)
	Procedures/surgeries
	Urgent care/emergency room visits
	Hospitalizations
	Primary medical and dental care (or lack thereof)
	Medication (including antibiotics during timeframe of concern)
	Immunizations (including hepatitis B and human papilloma virus)
Gynecologic history	Menstrual history
	Gender(s), age(s) of consensual partner(s), if any
	Contraceptive use

[a]Based on age of child and/or treating clinician's discretion
[b]Clearly indicate what was said by child, caregiver(s), or professional to treating clinician
[c]Questions should be limited in scope and relevant to current concerns, e.g., asking about consensual sexual activity only if within timeframe for collection of biological fluids in an acute assault

complete. In some cases, concern for child sexual abuse is the "chief complaint" as a result of disclosure to a family member, school official, or other mandated reporter. Disclosures that result in a formal investigation are most commonly made to mother (55%), grandmother (9%), or school official (7%) (Schaeffer, Leventhal, & Asnes, 2011). Young girls (age 7–13 years) are more likely to disclose immediately (in under a month) compared with older teenage girls; however, girls under 7 years at onset of abuse are least likely to disclose (Kogan, 2004). Younger children are more likely to tell adults (Schaeffer et al., 2011; Kogan, 2004). Older children are more likely to tell a peer; nearly half of teens are likely to initially disclose to a peer (Schaeffer et al., 2011; Kogan, 2004). Children may disclose sexual abuse because of their own adverse feelings or symptoms (e.g., anger, anxiety, and nightmares), factor(s) in the environment that facilitate disclosure, or after being questioned by a caregiver, teacher, or clinician (Schaeffer et al., 2011).

A disclosure of child sexual victimization is typically made weeks to years after event(s). Delayed disclosure and barriers to disclosure in childhood have been demonstrated in different populations. In a telephone survey of 804 Canadian adults, approximately 1 in 5 women and 1 in 10 men reported childhood sexual abuse. Of these individuals, 49% delayed disclosure by more than 5 years after the first episode, 21% never disclosed, and only 17% disclosed within 24 h (Hébert, Tourigny, Cyr, McDuff, & Joly, 2009). Canadian adult males disclosed at lower rates than females, with males more likely to not disclose at all; 34% of males and 16% females did not make a disclosure before the telephone survey. Barriers to disclosure in childhood include threats made by the perpetrator, fear of a caregiver's reaction and/or other ramifications of disclosure, and/or a child's lack of understanding about the experience (Schaeffer et al., 2011; Kogan, 2004). Among children who disclose, prepubescent boys disclose at a significantly lower rate than prepubescent girls (Heger, Ticson, Velasquez, et al., 2002b). A close and/or familial relationship with the perpetrator also reduces the likelihood of a disclosure (Schaeffer et al., 2011; Kogan, 2004).

Disclosures about child and adolescent sexual victimization are usually true although it is not the responsibility of the clinician to make this determination. False allegations are estimated to be in the 2–8% range (Everson & Boat, 1989). False recantations are also possible at a nonnegligible rate. Vaginal swabs and linen will sometimes test positive for sperm/semen in prepubescent children who deny ejaculation (Christian et al., 2000). Analysis of ten children's statements to police and videotaped episodes of their sexual abuse offer insight into factors that affect disclosure and recantation. Three to 23 months after videotaped episodes of sexual abuse, young children (mean age 6.9 years) may have difficulty remembering details, may be trying to forget or avoid details, or may simply prefer to not disclose (Sjöberg & Lindblad, 2002). Children may also not understand what happened and thus have difficulty sharing (Sjöberg & Lindblad, 2002). In this study of 102 videotaped episodes of sexual abuse, none of the children reported sexual abuse that was not documented on video (Sjöberg & Lindblad, 2002). Indeed, researchers concluded these young children minimized their experiences. Difficulty remembering details, trying to forget or avoid details, preferring not to disclose, or lack of understanding of victimization may also be inferred from other studies. Semen and/or sperm have been identified in instances when there are no disclosures of ejaculation by child victims evaluated after acute assault (Palusci, Cox, Shatz, & Schultze, 2006; Christian et al., 2000; Thackeray, Hornor, Benzinger, & Scribano, 2011).

Child sexual victimization is associated with psychological and behavioral difficulties in childhood that may continue to manifest in adulthood. Depression, posttraumatic stress disorder, substance use, sexual revictimization, and adverse parenting decisions are more likely in adult female survivors of child sexual victimization (Hornor, 2010). Linkage to community-based mental healthcare resources for the preschool-aged and older child and the non-offending caregiver is therefore the responsibility of the treating clinician. When a child is believed and supported by caregivers and clinicians, this can be an additional critical component in the child's psychological healing.

A clinician is mandated to make a report to CPS when there is reasonable suspicion of child sexual victimization. Statements made by caregiver(s) and/or child constitute reasonable suspicion of child sexual victimization. Many adults and some children realize information gathered during a medical encounter is shared among clinicians for purposes of diagnosis and treatment. If the history contains elements that are suspicious for child sexual victimization and/or other maltreatment, then the clinician should consider how and when to explain that information shared with a clinician in a case of suspected child sexual victimization is also divulged to social services and/or law enforcement professionals.

2.1.1 Obtaining a History from Caregiver(s)

The caregiver and the child should be spoken with separately when the clinician believes separation would not be detrimental. This allows the caregiver and clinician to share concerns that may not be appropriate for a child to overhear and/or may potentially influence a young child's disclosure (Jenny & Crawford-Jakubiak, 2013). The history of present illness (HPI) should include how abuse came to be suspected, including caregiver recall of prior concerning statements by the child and questions asked of the child by the caregiver (Jenny & Crawford-Jakubiak, 2013). **The HPI should include caregiver (and/or child's) statements about whether the child is believed by the principal caregiver(s).** A mother who asks the child (and not the abuser) whether the sexual abuse occurred, consistently believes the child, attributes the sexual abuse to the abuser, and is not a victim of intimate partner violence is more likely to protect the child from further harm (Coohey & O'Leary, 2008).

Caregivers may discuss adverse behaviors that indicate stress-induced dysregulation, including sexualized behavior exhibited by the child, when alone with the clinician. Sexualized behaviors may occur more frequently among sexually abused preteens compared with psychiatric patients without a history of sexual victimization and non-maltreated patients in some studies (Friedrich et al., 2001). Others note no relationship between the diagnosis of sexual abuse and sexualized behavior; rather that there is a correlation between sexualized behavior and mental health concerns (Drach, Wientzen, & Ricci, 2001). Sexually abused children do not consistently display sexualized behavior(s) (Drach et al., 2001). **The presence of sexualized behavior is not diagnostic of sexual abuse; rather, it is indicative of the need for mental health care.**

2.1.2 Obtaining a History from the Child

Children frequently perceive clinicians as individuals who can help by listening and treating their bodies. A child may use time alone with a clinician to discuss concerns or misconceptions the child may have about the child's body or health that may not have occurred to caregivers or clinicians. A medical history and/or review of systems before an examination allow a child to observe the clinician and the clinician to establish rapport with the child.

Before speaking with the child about possible maltreatment, it is best to establish that the clinician will ask questions to help with treatment of the child's body. Near the beginning of the encounter, the clinician might explain why and how she does check-ups, and for young children, discuss what the child believes happens when the child is at a doctor's office or hospital. If the clinician anticipates using equipment (camera, colposcope, ruler) that is not typically in a general practitioner's office, explaining the purpose of novel equipment alongside discussion about more traditional equipment (stethoscope, otoscope, etc.) with which the child may be familiar will help establish the clinical nature of the encounter. The clinician may then explain that even though she is a grown-up and a doctor or nurse she does not know everything that has happened to the child. The clinician must explicitly and repeatedly give the child permission to speak up, ask questions, voice assent to the examination process, and/or say the clinician is wrong or is not understood by the child.

Before asking questions about the event(s) that prompted formal medical care and/or the physical examination, the clinician must also explain to the child that the child is not in trouble with the doctor or nurse, and that the clinician will carefully listen to anything the child would like to share. Some clinicians also explain that what the child says and the words used by the child are important, and as such, the clinician may be writing or typing the child's words during their encounter.

A perfectly scripted medical encounter with a child is rare. Every child-serving clinician can share anecdotes about encounters that did not occur as planned. There will be times when the clinician walks into the exam room and has only just begun the process of introducing the clinician when the child begins to disclose the child's concerns. Disclosures about possible victimization may also occur during discussion about body safety after the examination, and during the review of systems. It is the clinician's responsibility to immediately begin to actively listen and look for signs, symptoms, and behavioral cues.

Clinicians must also remain aware of the child's development, particularly during history taking with the child. Clinician's comments and questions should ideally be short, simple, developmentally appropriate and/or open-ended (Table 2.2). **An open-ended approach ensures the clinician does not inadvertently suggest either abusive acts or a potential perpetrator to a young child. An open-ended approach also invites a child's narrative which may be replete with idiosyncratic comments, rich and unusual details.**

Taking a history from a verbal child outside of the presence of a caregiver allows the child to speak with the clinician without simultaneously observing and processing their caregiver's reactions. However, there are instances when either the caregiver or child does not feel separation is appropriate. Unless the child expresses another preference (e.g., to be in the lap of the caregiver), the caregiver may remain in the room but seated outside of the direct line of sight of the child when the clinician is speaking to the child.

An investigative or forensic interview sometimes occurs before the medical encounter. When this occurs, the clinician should make an effort to obtain details of the interview prior to examining the child to minimize repetition by the child and/or

Table 2.2 Suggestions for inviting narratives from a child

What	Tell me why you're getting a check-up today.
	Has something happened to your body that isn't ok?
	You can tell doctors/nurses anything that is true. What happened?
	I don't know what happened. Can you tell me?
	Tell me about a time you remember the most.
	You said [X]. Tell me what happened from beginning to end.
	What happened next?
	And then what happened?
	Tell me more about [X].
	What did you notice about your [body part] after [X]?
	What would you like to know about your body?
	What did [suspected perpetrator] say?
	What did [primary caregiver] say/do when you told?
Where	Where were your clothes?
	Where were perpetrator's clothes?
	Where were you [location] when [X] happened?
When	Did [X] happen one time or more than one time?
	Did [X] happen on one day or more than one day?
	When was the last time [X] happened?
	How old were you when [X] happened?
	Ask for details not a specific number.
Who	What is the name of the person who did [X] to you?
	What do grown-ups call [suspected perpetrator]?

[X] Child's words can be repeated back to child to invite further narrative or when clarification is needed

caregiver. Children may perceive repeated questions as being repeated because the adult does not approve of the child's response or does not believe the child's response is accurate. Nevertheless, even when the clinician has sufficient details about the events that raised concerns for sexual victimization, it remains important that the clinician consider speaking directly to the child. A medical history, review of systems and/or discussion about body safety may yield additional information, in addition to allowing the child to share the child's concerns.

Children who have experienced commercial sexual exploitation (CSE) have some characteristics that are different from child sexual abuse victims who have not experienced CSE (see Chap. 1). Male or female traffickers will sometimes pose as a caregiver, family friend, or paramour when the child presents for medical care. The child may also present with other trafficking victims. **Suspicion of trafficking is warranted when the person accompanying the child answers questions posed to the child, when the child lacks routine identification cards and/or is unfamiliar with their geographic location, particularly in the presence of additional risk factors for CSE in the history or on examination** (Greenbaum, Dodd, & McCracken, 2018). **A six-item screen has been developed to help identify children who experience commercial sexual exploitation:**

- Is there a previous history of drug and/or alcohol use?
- Has the youth ever run away from home?

- Has the youth ever been involved with law enforcement?
- Has the youth ever broken a bone, had traumatic loss of consciousness, or sustained a significant wound?
- Has the youth ever had a sexually transmitted infection?
- Does the youth have a history of sexual activity with more than five partners? (Greenbaum et al., 2018).

Children with two or more positive answers had nearly 22 times higher odds of being a CSE victim compared with a child with less than two positive responses (Greenbaum et al., 2018). Thought must be given to when and how to ask these CSE-related screening questions. The child must be separated from the adults or other children that accompany the child in a manner that does not arouse suspicion. Asking a child screening or other questions in a formal or direct fashion, or using a "checklist" approach, may not be ideal. Instead, interspersing screening questions with questions about the child's medical complaints may yield information.

2.2 Physical Examination

In addition to history taking, a careful and comprehensive physical examination can yield valuable information. The timing of a physical examination when sexual victimization is suspected depends on multiple factors (Table 2.3). A reasonable goal is a comprehensive medical examination, with or without forensic evidence collection, within days of disclosure or other evidence of sexual victimization. Consideration must be given to deferring an acute examination when it will negatively affect the child's mental health.

The physical examination should be done by or in consultation with available local experts such as Child Abuse Pediatricians. A comprehensive physical examination where the anogenital examination is simply one component of a holistic evaluation should be the clinician's goal. This conveys to the child that their overall health is important. Some clinicians deliberately conduct the anogenital component at the end of the exam. Other clinicians use a more traditional "head to toe" approach with the anogenital examination following the abdominal examination. A third option is to ask the child the order in which the child would like to be examined. A very young child will often spontaneously cue the clinician by reaching for an accessible stethoscope and placing it on their chest. This can be interpreted as engagement and/or assent and allows the exam to begin where the child is comfortable and familiar.

A comprehensive examination may reveal serious chronic medical concerns that have not been adequately treated such as signs of self-mutilation, dental decay, or asthma (Fig. 2.1). A comprehensive examination may reveal non-genital findings related to acute sexual abuse or assault such as intraoral injuries (petechiae, ecchymosis, frenulum injuries), bite marks inflicted by the suspected perpetrator, subtle

Table 2.3 Factors that may influence timing of medical examinations

Urgent (e.g., same day) examination	Mental health emergency (e.g., suicidal ideation)
	Acute genital or non-genital pain, bleeding, or injury
	Signs or symptoms of a sexually transmitted infection (STI)
	Meets criteria for HIV or other STI post-exposure prophylaxis
	Meets criteria for pregnancy prophylaxis
	Imminent danger or flight concerns (e.g., suspected human trafficking)
	Uncertainty about whether child will return for a scheduled examination
	Acute episode of sexual victimization with potential for transfer of biologic secretions
	Presentation within jurisdiction mandated time interval for forensic evidence collection
	Other unusual circumstances
Scheduled examination[a]	No emergency medical, mental health, or safety needs and outpatient clinic follow-up is likely
	Sexual victimization outside of mandated time interval for forensic evidence collection
	Sexualized behaviors and/or participation in developmentally inappropriate activities
	Concern for non-acute victimization in an asymptomatic child
	Another child in the household or other close child contact with an STI
	Need for linkage with community-based mental health and/or other resources
Second or follow-up examination[a]	Initial examination by an inexperienced clinician or clinician who requests a second opinion
	Equivocal findings (e.g., a potential medical mimic that cannot be ruled out with a single exam)
	STI testing not done during initial examination, or need for tests of cure
	Need for repeat testing for STIs or pregnancy (e.g., if prophylaxis was not offered or tolerated)

[a]Locations of nearest Child Advocacy Centers and/or Child Abuse Pediatricians in the United States and Canada can be found at https://www.aap.org/en-us/advocacy-and-policy/aap-health-initiatives/Child-Abuse-and-Neglect/Pages/State-Information-and-Resources-Map.aspx

signs of strangulation (hoarseness, subconjunctival hemorrhage, throat or neck pain), and cutaneous injuries (non-genital abrasions or bruises, tattoos) inflicted or facilitated by suspected perpetrator(s). Occasionally, a caregiver punishes the child because the caregiver believes the child is being untruthful about the sexual abuse or assault, resulting in cutaneous injuries. Areas of the body that are not being examined should be covered or gowned. Children should be allowed to opt out of all or part of the examination, particularly when they are asymptomatic.

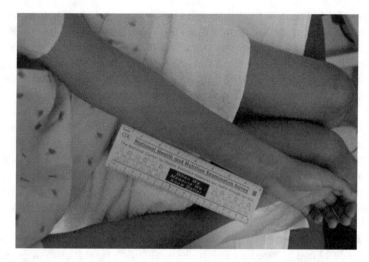

Fig. 2.1 Extragenital injuries. Teen with "runaway" episodes admitted to self-mutilation. She had multiple psychiatric hospitalizations before and after disclosing sexual abuse by father

2.2.1 Anogenital Exam

Careful and complete visualization of all external anogenital structures can be accomplished without increased trauma to the sexually victimized child. Psychological and physical distress before and during the anogenital examination can be minimized by educating and engaging both the child and caregiver(s). The examination, including anogenital examination, is reported to be less stressful than anticipated by both the caregiver and child with appropriate education (Marks, Lamb, & Tzioumi, 2009). Children are generally less distressed than their caregiver(s); further, the child's positive reaction generally has a calming effect on the caregiver(s) (Marks et al., 2009). Principles to minimize psychological stress include educating both the caregiver and child about the examination process and any procedures before the examination, specifically addressing with the child whether or not examination will involve injections or blood draws, involving the caregiver in the examination when possible, and addressing potential and actual embarrassment experienced by the child during the examination (Marks et al., 2009). Anecdotally, some clinicians also do extensive pre-examination teaching with caregivers, in part to minimize overt reactions or inopportune questions during the examination of the prepubescent child who generally prefers to have caregiver(s) present during their examination. Overall, a calm, unhurried approach with explanations and allowance for questions by the child and caregiver(s) is critical. At the end of the examination process, both parents and children typically express that clinician education and attitude and relationship between the clinician and child positively influenced their experience of the physical examination (Marks et al., 2009).

Areas of concern to the clinician during the anogenital exam are commonly described using the child's position (supine, prone, or left lateral decubitus)

and clock-face terminology. When referencing the female external genitalia and during the anogenital examination, 12 and 6 o'clock represent location of the midline structures. The numbers on the face of the clock are unchanged irrespective of the child's position. When supine, 3 o'clock refers to the child's left lateral hymen; when prone 3 o'clock refers to the right lateral hymen. Moving clockwise, the anterior hymen is between 10 and 2 o'clock. The posterior hymen is between 4 and 8 o'clock. In most cases, the anogenital examination begins in the supine position. In this position, there can be complete visualization of all of the external anogenital structures in prepubescent children and most males. In the *supine frog-leg* position, the legs and thighs of the young child are flexed and abducted while soles of feet are placed against each other as the child is resting on their back (Fig. 2.2). Taller prepubescent female children and female teens may be more comfortable in the *supine lithotomy* position with feet in stirrups. The perianal area can also be examined with the child supine and child's anterior thighs against their trunk.

The labia are separated by placing the gloved thumb and second fingers of the clinician's left hand between 8 and 9 o'clock on child's right labium majus and the thumb and second fingers of the clinician's right hand between 3 and 4 o'clock position on child's left labium majus. This is followed by *labial separation*: gentle lateral and downward separation of each labium. Labial separation can be followed by *labial traction*: gentle anterior traction towards clinician's body. Labia majora separation and/or traction usually result in complete visualization of the urethra and vaginal vestibule, particularly in prepubertal girls. In many instances, gentle, sustained traction on labia majora also results in the opening of the hymenal orifice (Fig. 2.3). During separation and traction in the prepubescent child, excessive manipulation of the less mobile labia minora should be avoided. Care must also be taken to avoid excessive tension on the skin of the posterior fourchette, which can cause discomfort in females of all ages. Touching and manipulation of the

Fig. 2.2 Supine frog-leg position

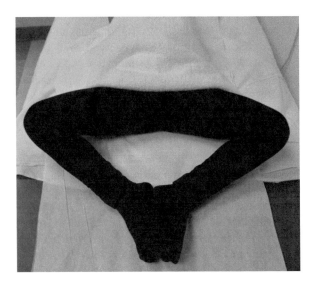

Fig. 2.3 Labial separation
and traction. Labia majora
(LMa) separation and
traction reveal annular
hymen (H) and
vaginal canal

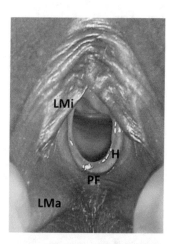

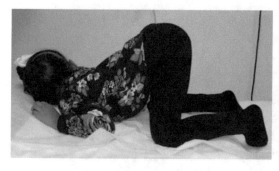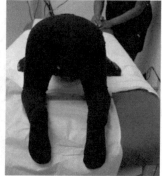

Fig. 2.4 Prone knee-chest position

unestrogenized, prepubescent hymen with a swab, speculum, or other object causes discomfort and anxiety in an alert prepubescent child and should be avoided.

Another useful examination position is the prone knee-chest position. (Fig. 2.4). In the prone knee-chest position, the child or teen is prone with their face and upper extremities on the examination table, abdomen down, back arched, buttocks raised above their back, thighs perpendicular to the examination table, and knees 6–8 inches apart. When the clinician's thumbs are placed near the base of the labia majora in prone knee-chest position (e.g., at 10 and 2 o'clock), sustained and steady upward pressure with clinician's thumbs generally allows for superior visualization of hymen, particularly the posterior hymen, along with the distal vaginal canal (Fig. 2.5).

The prone knee-chest position is extremely valuable when hymenal rim adherence or redundancy prevents complete visualization of the hymen when the child is supine. Figure 2.6 shows a hymen first in supine frog-leg position that appeared imperforate due to adherent hymenal edges; in prone knee-chest position, a normal annular hymen is visible. Prone knee-chest is also used to confirm suspected findings in or injuries to the posterior hymenal rim. Figure 2.7 exhibits a 15-year-old

Fig. 2.5 Visualization of hymen and distal vaginal canal in prone knee-chest position

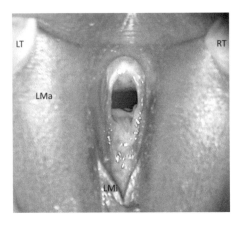

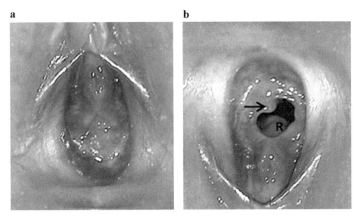

a   **b**

Fig. 2.6 Annular hymen. 10-year-old disclosed [male friend of mother] "touched me in all the wrong places with his hand." (**a**) Supine frog-leg position: hymen appeared imperforate due to adherent hymenal edges. (**b**) Prone knee-chest position: normal annular hymen. Mound abuts hymen at 10–11 o'clock. Intravaginal ridges (R) partially visible at 6 o'clock

with history of both consensual sexual contact and penile-vaginal assault. Figure 2.7a, taken in supine lithotomy, shows a possible hymenal transection at 6–7 o'clock. Figure 2.7b, in prone knee-chest position, confirms the transection at 12–1 o'clock. Prone knee-chest position allows for superior visualization of hymenal findings caused by penetrating sexual trauma (McCann, Voris, & Simon, 1992).

Improved visualization of the anus also occurs in the prone knee-chest position. In the prone knee-chest position, the anal sphincter(s) will dilate with, and sometimes without, clinician's gentle pressure on the area just around the perianal skin (Fig. 2.8) Despite these benefits, this examination position is not as frequently utilized in general practice compared with the supine examination position. Anecdotally, decreased familiarity with this position is one factor that increases clinician discomfort with the prone knee-chest position. However, neither the parent

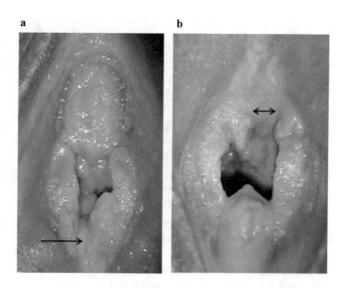

Fig. 2.7 Hymenal transection. 15-year-old with history of consensual sexual contact and penile-vaginal assault. (**a**) Supine lithotomy: possible hymenal transection at 6–7 o'clock. (**b**) Prone knee-chest position: transection (absence of hymenal tissue that extends the entire width of hymen to base) confirmed at 12–1 o'clock

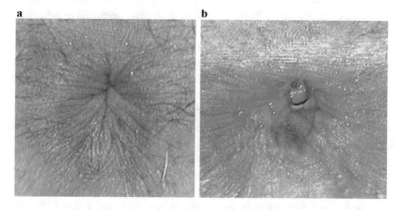

Fig. 2.8 (**a**) Closed external anal sphincter. Hyperpigmented perianal folds radiating from anal opening. Hyperpigmentation is a variation of normal skin pigment in children of color. (**b**) Partial reflex anal dilatation with lateral gluteal traction by examiner with child in prone knee-chest position

nor child finds this position to be a source of increased psychological stress with appropriate education (Marks et al., 2009). The disadvantage of the prone knee-chest position is the clinician cannot monitor the child's facial expression. Any examination position is potentially traumatic; therefore, if a caregiver or another clinician is available and appropriately prepared, that adult can stand close to the child to observe the child's facial expression and offer reassurance as needed.

Fig. 2.9 Perianal venous
congestion. Potentially
mimics bruising. Flattened
anal folds may be caused
by relaxation of the anal
sphincter or swelling due
to trauma

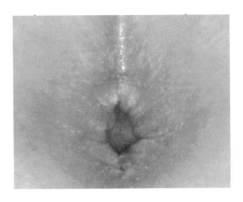

It should be noted that sustained examination, particularly in the prone knee-chest position, can result in dependent pooling of blood and temporary obstruction of venous outflow. This dependent pooling of blood gives the perianal skin a bluish discoloration which should not be mistaken for bruising (Fig. 2.9). Discoloration quickly resolves with a change in position and/or ambulation.

Some males prefer to stand rather than be examined in prone knee-chest position. Standing allows for access to the penis and scrotum. As an alternative to the prone knee-chest position, the anus can be examined with the child in the left lateral decubitus position. In the left lateral decubitus position, the child is asked to place their anterior thighs against or as close as possible to their chest. The examiner then performs lateral traction with each gloved hand parallel to child's gluteal cleft.

In addition to careful positioning of the patient, other examination methods may be utilized to evaluate for potential trauma. Estrogen causes a thickened, redundant hymen (Fig. 2.10). In pubertal patients with estrogenized hymens, a swab can be used to assess the continuity of a thickened, redundant hymenal rim (Fig. 2.11). Among female teens who are Tanner III or above, use of a Foley bladder catheter to evaluate the hymenal rim is an alternative to the prone knee-chest position and/or tracing of the hymenal rim with a swab. Two clinicians, a 12- or 14-gauge Foley bladder catheter with a 5- to 10-cc balloon and a 10-cc syringe filled with water are needed (Starling & Jenny, 1997). The catheter is inserted into the vaginal canal. The balloon is then filled to capacity with 10 cc of water and the syringe removed. One clinician performs labial traction while the second clinician retracts the catheter until the balloon is in contact with the hymen. This reduces hymenal redundancy. The catheter is then moved to the right then left causing the balloon to delineate the left then right hymenal rim (Starling & Jenny, 1997). Once there is adequate visualization of the hymenal rim, the balloon is deflated and withdrawn. **During the assessment of sexually victimized pediatric patients, a speculum or scope is rarely used. Prepubescent patients are generally sedated before the use of a speculum or scope.** A speculum or scope may be indicated when there is concern for internal trauma such as vaginal wall or intestinal injuries, or foreign bodies that are not in the anterior vaginal canal.

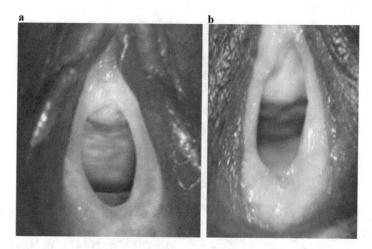

Fig. 2.10. (a) Relatively translucent annular hymen with visualization of blood vessels. Then 7-year-old Tanner I female disclosed fondling by step-father. (b) Thickened hymen. Now 13-year-old Tanner III female (first seen as a 7-year-old in Fig. 2.10a) disclosed penile-vaginal contact with brother

2.2.2 Variations of Normal Anogenital Anatomy

There is a wide range of normal anatomical variants and few anogenital findings that are definitive physical evidence of penetrating sexual trauma. The hymen is tissue that rims and partially covers the vaginal orifice. It has no known physiologic function, but often is of tremendous psychological and cultural importance. In the absence of major anogenital abnormalities, all newborn girls have hymens (Jenny, Kuhns, & Arakawa, 1987; Berenson, 1995). A normal hymen can have multiple configurations: annular, crescentic, fimbriated, sleeve-like, septate, cribriform, and microperforate. Annular and crescentic hymens are the most common configurations (Myhre, Berntzen, & Bratlid, 2003; Heger, Ticson, Guerra, et al., 2002a; Berenson et al., 2000). An annular hymen has a continuous rim with relatively even amounts of hymenal tissue anteriorly (between 9 and 3 o'clock) and posteriorly (between 3 o'clock and 9 o'clock). (Figs. 2.6, 2.11, 2.15, 2.21, 2.25, 2.30, and 2.34). A crescentic hymen has no hymenal tissue between 11 and 1 o'clock with a relatively abundant posterior rim that can vary in width (Figs. 2.16, 2.20, and 2.35b). A fimbriated hymen has a scalloped appearance created by multiple superficial notches (partial clefts). Notches (clefts) are U- or V-shaped indentations in the hymenal rim that can be superficial (less than or equal to half of the hymenal rim) (Fig. 2.11) or deep (more than half but not extending to the base of the hymen). A sleeve hymen has rolled, usually thickened, edges that may largely obscure the hymenal opening (Fig. 2.12). A septate hymen has two hymenal openings caused by a diagonal band of tissue that partially obscures a single vaginal canal (Fig. 2.13). A hymen can also have no hymenal opening (imperforate) (Fig. 2.14), a single very small opening (microperforate), or multiple very small openings (cribriform). An imperforate

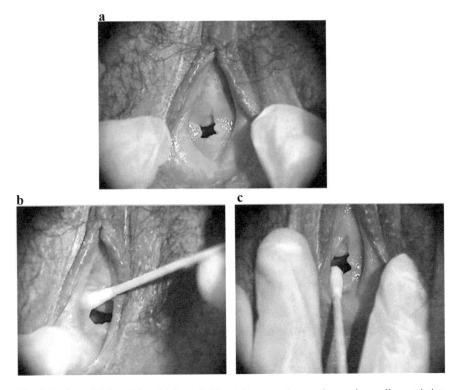

Fig. 2.11 Superficial notching. (**a**) Superficial notching anywhere on hymen is usually a variation of normal anatomy. (**b**) Swab is used to evaluate continuity of hymenal rim. (**c**) Superficial notch at 3 o'clock

Fig. 2.12 Sleeve-like hymen. Labia minora (LMi) and urethra (U) also visible in addition to estrogenized hymen (H)

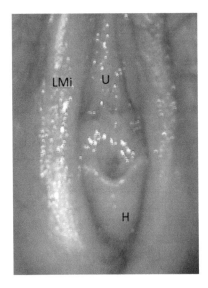

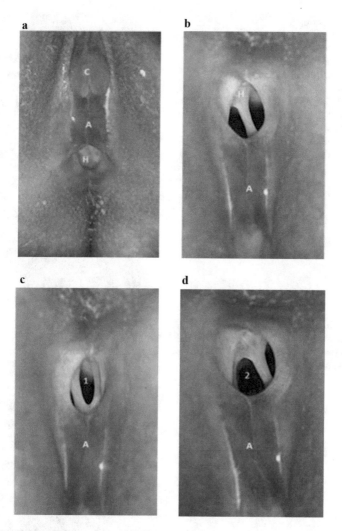

Fig. 2.13 (**a**) Labial adhesions. Anterior labial adhesions (A) largely obscure hymen when patient supine. Clitoral hood (C) also visible. (**b**) Septum of hymen creating two hymenal orifices seen in prone knee-chest position. (**c**) First (1) hymenal orifice. (**d**) Second (2) hymenal orifice

hymen is a congenital anomaly. The urethral and/or hymenal orifices can be partially or completely obscured by labial adhesion(s). A labial adhesion is caused by fusion of the adjacent edges of the labia minora; adhesion(s) can occur anteriorly (Fig. 2.13a) or posteriorly along the length of the vaginal vestibule.

In addition to various normal hymenal configurations, there are associated hymenal features that are variations of normal hymenal and anogenital anatomy. Each of the following variants has been seen in newborn females and/or populations of girls not believed to have been abused: urethral dilatation with labial traction (Fig. 2.15), vestibular (periurethral or perihymenal) bands (Fig. 2.16), prominent

Fig. 2.14 Imperforate
hymen. 6-year-old seen
after anonymous CPS
report of abnormal
genitalia. Imperforate
hymen when supine
(shown) and in prone
knee-chest. At age 8 years,
a microperforation
developed without surgical
intervention (not shown)

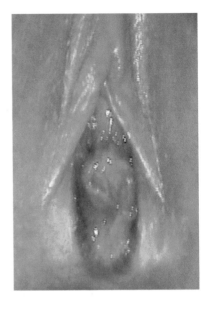

Fig. 2.15 Urethral and
hymenal dilatation. Supine
with labia majora
separation and traction

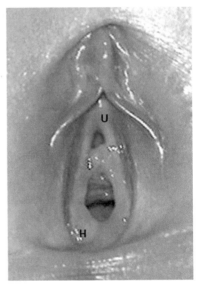

hymenal vessels (Fig. 2.10a), hymenal tags, hymenal mounds (bumps) (Fig 2.6b),
superficial hymenal notches (clefts) (Figs. 2.11), narrow hymens with smooth continuous rims (Fig. 2.3), longitudinal intravaginal ridges (Fig. 2.17), and linea vestibularis (Berenson, 1995; Heger, Ticson, Guerra, et al., 2002a; Myhre et al., 2003).
Vestibular (periurethral or perihymenal) bands are lateral to either the urethra or
hymen and connect to the walls of the vaginal vestibule (Fig. 2.16). Hymenal tags
are elongated protrusions of hymenal tissue. Hymenal mounds (bumps) are

Fig. 2.16 Vestibular
bands. Periurethral or
perihymenal bands (B)
must not be mistaken for
scarring

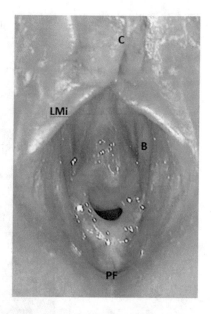

Fig. 2.17 Longitudinal
Intravaginal Ridges

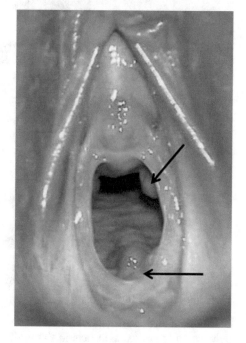

sometimes caused by longitudinal intravaginal ridges abutting the hymen (Fig. 2.6b).
Hymenal mounds can occur in isolation. Finally, linea vestibularis is a midline, flat,
avascular area found below the hymen in the posterior fossa of girls selected for
non-abuse (Kellogg & Parra, 1991).

Fig. 2.18 Perianal skin tag. Anterior to anal opening (12 o'clock) in a torture survivor. A similar proportion of children with penetrating anal trauma and non-abused children have a midline perianal skin tag

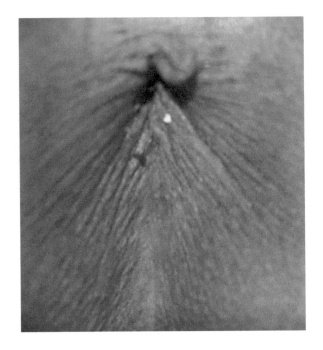

Fig. 2.19 Hymenal petechiae (4 o'clock)

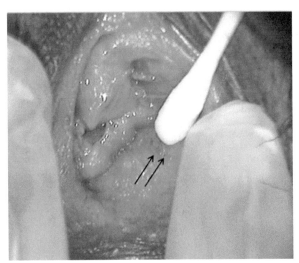

Some of these variants of normal anogenital anatomy, in particular hymenal notches and perianal skin tags in the midline, can also be the sequelae of trauma (Heppenstall-Heger et al., 2003; McCann, Miyamoto, Boyle, & Rogers, 2007a; McCann & Voris, 1993). Superficial hymenal notches in both the anterior and posterior hymen have been noted in prepubertal children not suspected to have been sexually abused (Heger, Ticson, Guerra, et al., 2002a). However, acute hymenal

Fig. 2.20 Hymenal
bruising (2–5 o'clock)

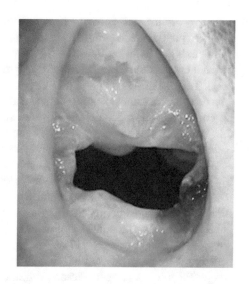

injuries that are followed over time may heal in a manner that creates the appearance of a superficial notch (McCann, Miyamoto, Boyle, & Rogers, 2007b; McCann et al., 1992; Heppenstall-Heger et al., 2003). Similarly, although a perianal skin tag is often regarded as a variant of normal anogenital anatomy, a perianal laceration that extends to the anal verge may heal with a residual perianal skin tag in the midline (Heppenstall-Heger et al., 2003; McCann & Voris, 1993 (Fig. 2.18). The physical examination, whether normal or abnormal, must thus be interpreted in the context of historical and/or behavioral factors, a psychosocial assessment, and a law enforcement investigation. In isolation, none of the variations of normal anogenital anatomy should be attributed to trauma, particularly if an acute injury was not previously documented in the same location. Conversely, penetrating sexual trauma injury may in rare cases manifest in an unusual manner. For instance, an imperforate hymen is usually an isolated congenital abnormality. It is usually asymptomatic and of no clinical significance until puberty when menstrual flow is obstructed. However, an imperforate hymen may in rare cases be acquired as a result of scar tissue formation following a sexual assault with significant injuries in a prepubescent child (Botash & Jean-Louis, 2001). Thus, an imperforate hymen does not rule out the possibility of sexual trauma, including penetrating sexual trauma (Botash & Jean-Louis, 2001).

2.2.3   Hymenal Injuries

Acute injuries are most likely to be detected in pre- and post-pubertal girls examined within 7 days of sexual victimization (Watkeys, Price, Upton, & Maddocks, 2008). Petechiae (Fig. 2.19), bruising (Fig. 2.20), abrasions, and lacerations are indicative of acute, blunt force hymenal trauma. More often, a clinician is tasked with interpreting non-acute or healed findings. **Superficial and deep hymenal notches (partial clefts) must be distinguished from hymenal transections (complete clefts).** A hymenal transection (complete cleft) is a concavity in the hymenal rim that extends the entire width of the hymen to the hymenal base (Figs. 2.7 and 2.21). The distinction among these three entities is typically made by use of more than one examination technique; supine examination followed by confirmation with (a) prone knee-chest positioning, (b) tracing of the hymen with a swab, and/or (c) foley catheter. Deep hymenal notches and hymenal transections between 4 and 8 o'clock have only been described in prepubertal girls with a history of vaginal penetration (Berenson et al., 2000; Heppenstall-Heger et al., 2003). **A transection in the posterior hymen (between 4 and 8 o'clock) is consistent with healed penetrating, blunt force trauma, including sexual trauma** (Berkoff et al., 2008; Adams, Farst, & Kellogg, 2018). Anogenital findings occur more frequently in pubertal children with a history of penetrating trauma (Adams, Botash, & Kellogg, 2004; Al-Jilaihawi et al., 2017). Sexually transmitted infections, a disclosure of penetrating trauma, and assault by a non-biological parent increase the likelihood of anogenital injuries (Heger, Ticson, Velasquez, et al., 2002b). History of bleeding with abuse also increases the likelihood of abnormal anogenital findings (Anderst, Kellogg, & Jung, 2009; Adams, Harper, Knudson, & Revilla, 1994).

2.2.4 Anal and Other Non-Hymenal Injuries

Parents and investigators will ask multiple questions about the appearance and integrity of the hymen. It is the clinician's responsibility not to overlook evidence of trauma or other pathology involving the anus and other non-hymenal structures. A penile frenulum tear, bite marks, bruises, and/or lesions are possible penile injuries. Bruising, fissures, lacerations, edema, and rare scars may be noted to the labia, vestibule, posterior fourchette, posterior fossa, perineum, and/or anus (Figs. 2.22, 2.23, and 2.24) Among 23 children, age 16 years or younger, who provided a history of penetrating anal trauma and were examined within 7 days of the last event, 56% (13 children) were noted to have anal and perianal findings: bruising (7 children), lacerations (6 children), and/or an anal scar (1 child) (Watkeys et al., 2008). Among 198 children (mean age 9 years), 47% of whom were examined within 72 h of probable anal penetration, approximately 15.3% (30 children) were noted to have anal fissures or lacerations, 2% (4 children) were noted to have bruising, and no children had perianal scaring (Myhre et al., 2013). Probably anal penetration was defined by historical details, adult witness observations, forensic evidence, photographic evidence, or presence of gonorrhea (Myhre et al., 2013). Total anal dilatation (dilatation of both external and internal sphincters with visualization into the rectum) was documented in 12.1% of children believed to have probable anal penetration compared with 3.6% of controls ($p < 0.05$) (Myhre et al., 2013). Despite this significant difference between victims and controls in this latter study, others have cautioned

Fig. 2.21 Hymenal transection (4 o'clock)

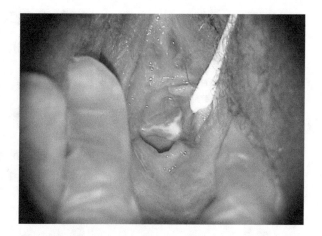

Fig. 2.22 Perianal fissures. 14-year-old disclosed penile-anal assault 12 h before exam. Perianal fissures (between 4 and 7 o'clock) on prone knee-chest exam. Perianal fissures can be caused by penetrating sexual contact, constipation, and infections

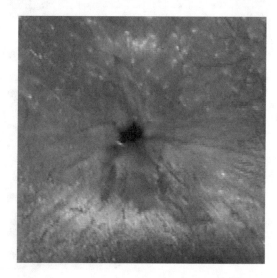

there is insufficient literature and lack of consensus about the significance and association of complete anal dilatation with penetrating anal trauma (Adams et al., 2018).

2.2.5 Interpreting Anogenital Findings (or Lack Thereof): The Normalcy of a Normal Anogenital Exam

A normal examination does not mean that sexual victimization has not occurred. Understanding and discussing clinician, caregiver, and investigator expectations that there should be acute or healed hymenal and/or other anogenital injuries following child sexual victimization is an important aspect of the medical

Fig. 2.23 Posterior fossa lacerations. 15-year-old with dysuria and vaginal pain hours after penile-vaginal assault. Estrogenized hymen (H) showed no acute injury

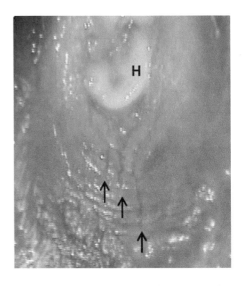

Fig. 2.24 Multiple acute perianal injuries. 2-year-old with anogenital bleeding suspected to have been sexually assaulted by mother's boyfriend. Perianal bruising (B), edema (E), and lacerations (arrows) resulted in loss of perianal skin folds and poor sphincter tone

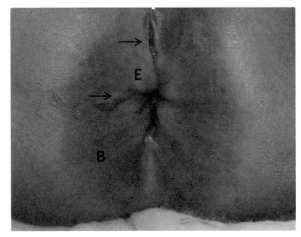

evaluation. Some older children and caregivers express the false belief that clinicians and others can look at their genitalia and know whether there was penetration of the vaginal or anal orifices. **In reality, the anogenital examination of the sexually abused prepubescent child is usually not different from the child not believed to be sexually abused** (Berenson et al., 2000). Less than 7% of all children referred for medical examinations following suspected sexual victimization will have abnormal examination findings (Al-Jilaihawi et al. 2017; Smith, Raman, Madigan, Waldman & Shouldice, 2018; Gallion et al., 2016; Heger, Ticson, Guerra, et al., 2002a; Berenson et al., 2000). Similarly, teens who admit to consensual and non-consensual sexual contact, and some pregnant teens, have been noted to have

Fig. 2.25 Superficial (partial) hymenal notch (10 o'clock). Pregnant 13-year-old without definitive hymenal injury disclosed penile-vaginal penetration by uncle. Similar partial notches in the anterior hymen are noted in girls selected for non-abuse (Berenson et al., 2000)

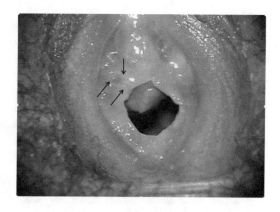

similar, normal hymenal findings (Adams et al., 2004; Anderst et al., 2009) (Fig. 2.25). "It's normal to be normal" (Adams et al., 1994).

Definitive physical findings of anogenital trauma (acute lacerations, abrasions, petechiae, bruising, healed hymenal transections, and anogenital scarring) are only seen in a minority of child victims (Adams et al., 2018). Normal anogenital examinations have been documented following multiple episodes of penetrating sexual trauma (Anderst et al., 2009). There are several reasons why an anogenital examination is most likely to be normal following one or more episodes of penetrating sexual trauma, including:

1. **The hymen is recessed compared to labia majora and minora and posterior fourchette.** There may be labial but not hymenal or vaginal canal penetration by an object, finger, or penis during episode(s) of sexual victimization. Young children may describe contact between and posterior to the labia majora to be inside the vagina (Heger, Ticson, Guerra, et al., 2002a; Anderst et al., 2009; Gallion et al., 2016). Similarly, there may be gluteal cleft but not anal orifice penetration.

2. **Physical injury may or may not occur depending on the size of penetrating object relative to stretching and distention of the vaginal or anal orifice.** Penile-vaginal penetration is associated with more significant injuries and likelihood of complete hymenal transections compared with digital-vaginal penetration (Heppenstall-Heger et al., 2003).

3. **Injuries may be overlooked or misinterpreted.** This can occur depending on level of relaxation or cooperation of the child, and/or experience of the clinician with use of various examination techniques. The prone knee-chest position allows for superior visualization of posterior hymenal findings caused by penetrating sexual trauma (McCann et al., 1992).

4. **Most anogenital injuries heal quickly and completely, and typically without scarring** (McCann et al., 1992; Heppenstall-Heger et al., 2003). Anogenital petechiae, ecchymosis, edema, and abrasions resolve quickly, usually within

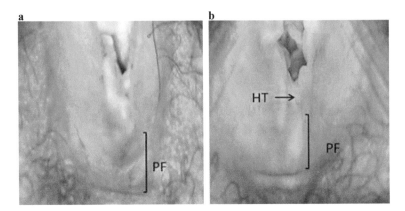

Fig. 2.26 (**a**) Posterior fossa abrasions. 16-year-old disclosed penile-vaginal assault 1 day before initial exam. (**b**) Resolution of abrasions noted 3 days after assault on follow-up exam. Incidental healed hymenal transection (HT, at 6 o'clock, not attributed to acute assault) on initial and follow-up exams

5 days (McCann et al., 2007a, 2007b) (Fig. 2.26). A perianal laceration that extends to the anal verge usually heals without residual scarring, or with nonspecific perianal skin fold changes including a perianal skin tag (Heppenstall-Heger et al., 2003; McCann & Voris, 1993) (Fig. 2.27). Partial hymenal transections in children of all ages heal completely or heal with a residual notch or mild irregularity that could be interpreted as normal if not seen acutely (McCann et al., 2007a; Heppenstall-Heger et al., 2003). A complete hymenal transection may not heal completely without surgical intervention; complete healing is possible with surgical intervention (Heppenstall-Heger et al., 2003). Scarring and pigmentary changes are typically only seen following a deep laceration to non-hymenal structures and/or surgical repair of non-hymenal structures (Heppenstall-Heger et al., 2003; McCann & Voris, 1993).

5. **Disclosure of child sexual victimization is often delayed. Passage of time is correlated with decreased likelihood of finding anogenital injuries** (Adams et al., 1994). In one study of girls aged 3–8 years, the median length of time from the last episode of digital or penile sexual abuse to examination was 42 days. In this study, less than 5% of vaginal examinations were abnormal (Berenson et al., 2000).

6. **Estrogen, in infants or teens, causes the hymen to become thick and/or redundant**. This may prevent the examiner from immediately recognizing the extent of acute hymenal injuries or obscure residue of non-acute hymenal injuries (McCann et al., 1992, 2007b).

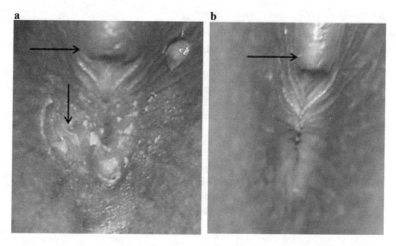

Fig. 2.27 (**a**) Healing perianal laceration. 7-year-old with sexualized behavior had painful, bloody bowel movement 5 days before note of a healing laceration (vertical arrow) with surrounding swelling on initial exam. (**b**) Repigmentation. Healing and complete repigmentation 8 days later (13 days after initial complaint). Incidental diastasis ani (horizontal arrows), a normal congenital variant

2.3 Differential Diagnosis and "Mimics" of Sexual Trauma

Children may present with anogenital complaints and findings which may potentially mimic injuries caused by sexual abuse or assault (see Table 2.4). Medical conditions and child sexual victimization can of course co-exist. Therefore, the mere presence of intrinsic pathology does not mean sexual victimization has not occurred. Careful history taking and physical examination(s) often help distinguish among possible diagnoses and mimics.

Anogenital bleeding and/or bruising can be caused by nonsexual accidental trauma in a manner that may mimic acute sexual abuse or assault. Bleeding and/or bruising can be due to straddle injury (most common), non-straddle blunt trauma, and penetrating trauma (Iqbal et al., 2010). **Typical straddle injuries among females involve the external genitalia and/or structures anterior to the relatively recessed hymen** (Fig. 2.30). Independently mobile girls who sustain straddle injuries most often have unilateral labial and clitoral hood injuries. Accidental penetrating injuries and injuries to the hymen are uncommon (8.4%) forms of accidental, anogenital trauma (Iqbal et al., 2010). Male children may have penile entrapment with zippers and toilet seats, along with perineal and scrotal trauma associated with direct blunt trauma during sports. The spectrum of motor vehicular crush injuries (in children run over by slow-moving vehicles) occasionally includes multiple anogenital abrasions and bruises, vaginal, hymenal, and/or perianal lacerations (Boos, Rosas, Boyle, & McCann, 2003). These children with anogenital injuries due to the motor vehicular crush mechanism also have injuries to the skin, abdomen, and/or pelvis (Boos et al., 2003).

Table 2.4 Anogenital Mimics of Sexual Trauma

Predominant findings	Differential diagnosis
Bleeding	Accidental trauma Straddle (Fig. 2.30) injuries Non-straddle blunt trauma Penetrating trauma Motor vehicular/crush injuries Dehisced labial adhesions Lichen sclerosus Infection (e.g., *Shigella flexneri*) Urethral polyps Urethral prolapse (Fig. 2.31) Urinary tract infection Vaginal foreign body Anal fissure(s) Hemorrhoids Crohn's disease Rectal prolapse Precocious puberty Vaginal or cervical tumors
Bruising	Lichen sclerosus (Fig. 2.32) Hemangioma(s) (vulva, urethra, hymen) Henoch-Schonlein purpura (penis, scrotum, buttocks) Perianal venous congestion (Fig. 2.9)
Erythema	Irritant contact dermatitis Soaps, bubble baths, shampoos, bleach Prolonged contact with urine, feces, moisture Infections *Streptococcus pyogenes* (group A streptococcus) *Staphylococcus aureus*
Vaginal discharge	Infections including *Streptococcus pyogenes* (group A streptococcus) *Streptococcus agalactiae* (group B streptococcus) *Staphylococcus aureus* *Hemophilus influenzae* *Shigella flexneri* (often bloody) *Gardnerella vaginalis* *Escherichia coli* *Candida* *Enterobius vermicularis* (pinworms) Vaginal foreign bodies Exudate (from healing accidental trauma) Physiologic leucorrhea Precocious puberty Tumors Exogenous estrogen
Ulcers	Normal variants Midline fusion defects Diastasis ani (Fig. 2.27) Infections Varicella zoster Epstein-Barr virus Behcet's syndrome

(continued)

Table 2.4   (continued)

Predominant findings	Differential diagnosis
Papules and nodules	Normal variants
	Periurethral cysts
	Skin tags
	Pink pearly penile papules
	Infections
	Human papillomavirus
	Molluscum contagiosum
	Folliculitis
	Pediculosis pubis
	Scabies
	Pseudoverrucous papules and nodules (Fig. 2.28)
	Sarcoma botryoides (intravaginal nodules or protruding mass)
Scarring	Labial adhesions
	Asymmetric vestibular (periurethral and perihymenal) bands
	Linea vestibularis
	Prominent median raphe
	Crohn's Disease (Fig. 2.29)
	Medical/surgical interventions

Adapted from *Child Abuse and Neglect: Diagnosis, Treatment, and Evidence* by C. Jenny 2011, Saunders/Elsevier, St. Louis, MO

Fig. 2.28 Pseudoverrucous papules and nodules. 8-year-old obese female with chronic urinary incontinence made no concerning disclosures. Smooth, flat, round lesions (usually 2–8 mm) are an irritant reaction to prolonged exposure to urine and/or stool. Suprapubic and perianal lesions are also possible. Appearance may mimic anogenital warts

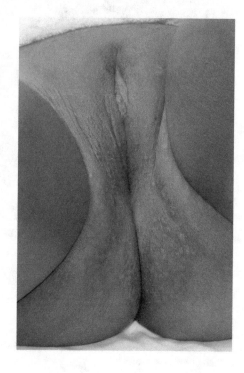

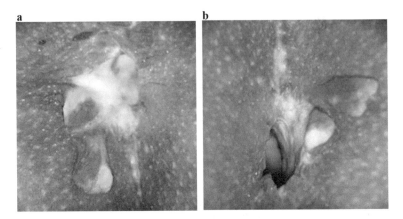

Fig. 2.29 Crohn's Disease. 14-year-old with Crohn's Disease disclosed non-acute penile-vaginal assault. Her vaginal exam was normal. (**a**) Supine: Large, hard perianal skin tags. Distorted perianal tissue. (**b**) Prone knee-chest: Complete anal dilatation. In addition to skin tags (1–3 o'clock), perianal fissures, fistulas, and abscesses and vulvitis are possible disease complications

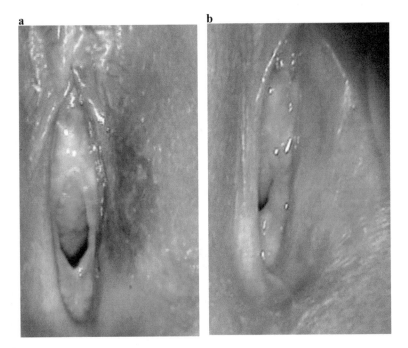

Fig. 2.30 Straddle injury. 10-year-old on bicycle with another girl when they fell. Child made no concerning disclosures. (**a**) Vaginal pain prompted exam on day of fall. Note unilateral nature of injuries. Recessed hymen is unaffected. (**b**) Labium minus and vestibular ecchymosis resolved by second exam 4 days later

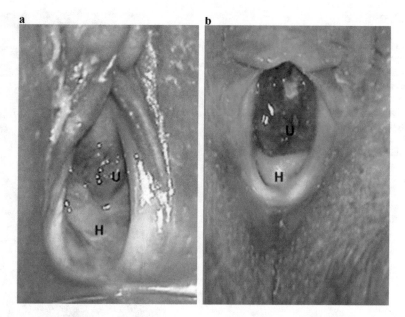

Fig. 2.31 Urethral prolapse. Most commonly seen in prepubescent African-American children. (**a**) Asymptomatic protruding urethra (U) in a child with constipation. She disclosed physical abuse. (**b**) Bleeding, bright red tissue largely obscuring hymen (H) noted after complaints of possible straddle injury, vaginal bleeding, and dysuria in a second child

Urethral prolapse can present with bleeding, typically following accidental trauma, and may mimic acute hymenal injury. Urethral prolapse also presents incidentally as a protruding mass, often in a prepubertal child with a history of constipation. Sometimes, the hymen is partially obscured by the prolapsed urethra (Fig. 2.31). A cotton swab can be used to elevate the prolapsed tissue and expose the hymen. Preferably, prolapsed urethral tissue can be differentiated from the hymen when the child assumes the prone knee-chest position. **Urethral prolapse may occasionally be confused with a large wart caused by human papillomavirus, a urethral hemangioma, or may mimic Sarcoma botryoides (a genital tract rhabdomyosarcoma that usual presents as a protruding intravaginal mass).** Consultation with a urologist and/or pediatric gynecologist is often helpful.

Lichen sclerosus is characterized by hypopigmented, atrophic, and friable skin that may bleed with trauma. Lichen sclerosus is most commonly noted on the vulva, glans penis, perineum, and/or perianal skin of prepubescent children (Fig. 2.32). Even minimal trauma may result in fissuring, submucosal hemorrhage, and hematomas. Alternatively, the child may complain of itching and dysuria which prompts close inspection of the anogenital region and identification of abnormal skin findings.

Fig. 2.32 Lichen sclerosus. Seen more often in prepubescent children compared with teens. 8-year-old with several weeks of vaginal itching made no concerning disclosures. White, atrophic skin noted on clitoral hood, labia minora, medial aspect of labia majora, and perineum. Submucosal hemorrhage is noted on right labia minus, labia majora, and posterior fossa

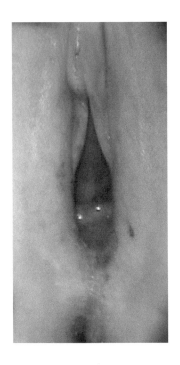

In addition to concerns about bleeding and bruising, any cutaneous midline finding(s) should be cautiously analyzed as midline finding(s) may both mimic or be caused by acute and non-acute sexual and physical trauma. Linea vestibularis is a midline, flat, avascular area found below the hymen in the posterior fossa of girls selected for non-abuse (Kellogg & Parra, 1991). Linea vestibularis may be difficult to differentiate from scarring, although scarring is classically raised or irregular and more easily diagnosed if an acute injury was previously documented in the same location. Midline fusion defects are also possible mimics. These include congenital failure of midline fusion (perineal groove), infantile pyramidal protrusion, prominent median raphe, and diastasis ani (McCann, Voris, Simon, & Wells, 1989). An infantile pyramidal protrusion is a smooth red or pink protrusion of tissue in the midline anterior to the anus. A median raphe is a prominent, often hyperpigmented ridge in the midline of the perineum. Diastasis ani refers to the absence of muscle fibers in the midline of the external anal sphincter which creates a fan-shaped loss of anal folds in the midline (Fig. 2.27). These midline fusion defects show no evidence of scarring. **Serial examinations help with the distinction between a congenital midline defect and trauma; the midline fusion defect will not undergo short-term changes. Indeed, serial examinations generally help with differentiation among anogenital trauma and many potential mimics.**

2.4 Forensic Examination

In most jurisdictions in the United States, forensic evidence collection is generally recommended for all children who present within 72 h of sexual victimization that has the potential for physical transfer of biologic secretions. In teen and adult sexual assault victims, there appears to be little variability in the microscopic detection of sperm and detection of physical injuries over this timeframe (Ingemann-Hansen, Brink, Sabroe, Sørensen, & Charles, 2008). In the prepubescent population, a forensic examination performed within 24 h of the assault is most likely to yield identifiable DNA and trace evidence (Girardet et al., 2011; Christian et al., 2000; Thackeray et al., 2011; Palusci et al., 2006). Identifiable DNA has occasionally been collected from body swabs after 24 h has elapsed since the sex crime was perpetrated on a pubescent child (Girardet et al., 2011; Thackeray et al., 2011). However, outside of the 24-hour timeframe, forensic evidence is most likely to be found on clothing and bed linen rather than on swabs collected from body surfaces and orifices of prepubescent children (Christian et al., 2000; Palusci et al., 2006; Girardet et al., 2011). Complete DNA profiles can be obtained from laundered clothing 8 months after semen deposition (Brayley-Morris et al., 2015). Factors associated with positive evidence collection and DNA detection are a history of perpetrator ejaculation and genital to genital contact (Thackeray et al., 2011; Palusci et al., 2006). However, identifiable DNA, semen, and/or sperm has been occasionally collected in instances of normal examination findings, when there was no reported ejaculation, and in cases of fondling without reported ejaculation (Palusci et al., 2006; Christian et al., 2000; Thackeray et al., 2011; Girardet et al., 2011). Bleeding and visible injuries increase the likelihood of forensic evidence recovery in prepubescent children (Christian et al., 2000). Female gender, positive/abnormal examination findings, age greater than 10 years, puberty, and perpetrator aged 15 years or older also predict positive forensic examinations (Palusci et al., 2006). As many as 82% of prepubescent children with normal anogenital or nonspecific examination findings have DNA evidence from body swabs (Girardet et al., 2011).

Forensic evidence collection kits are self-contained with fairly standard instructions for clinicians across most jurisdictions in the United States (Fig. 2.33). In some jurisdictions within the United States, forensic kits are readily available at medical facilities. In other jurisdictions, a forensic kit is provided by law enforcement after a preliminary investigation. Collection of biologic secretions (blood or saliva of a perpetrator, semen, sperm) and trace evidence is ideally done at the same time as the acute medical examination. Medical or surgical treatment of acute injuries should not be delayed for an inordinate amount of time because of clinician's fear of evidence destruction or contamination. In addition to the contents of the kit, the clinician will need to have a change of clothing for the child, ruler or measuring tape, photographic and/or colposcopic equipment, and multiple pairs of gloves available in a private examination room. A plan for drying wet evidence and/or handling wet items (wet clothing, sanitary pads, tampons, diapers) during evidence collection is essential. Wet items should be stored in paper (never plastic) bags and

Fig. 2.33 Forensic
evidence collection:
self-contained kit typically
contains instructions,
consent and documentation
forms, paper bags for
clothing, collection paper
for debris, comb for pubic
hair combing, swabs,
and smears

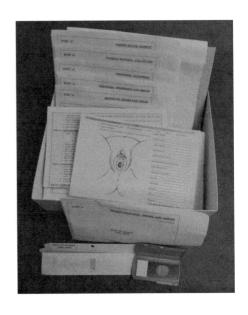

refrigerated to minimize the growth of bacteria or fungus. A child often also appreciates being able to sip on juice and have access to wipes and sanitary napkins as soon as possible after appropriate swabs are obtained, even if their examination has not yet ended.

In the United States, the Violence Against Women Reauthorization Act of 2013 (2013) and Survivors' Bill of Rights Act of 2016 (2016) ensures clinicians discuss several rights with children and/or their caregivers. Children and caregivers need to be aware that a forensic examination and medical treatment can occur following an acute event, all or some components of the examination can be refused, forensic evidence will be stored at the medical facility whether or not law enforcement is involved, forensic evidence will be turned over to law enforcement based on family's wishes, and there will be no charge for the forensic examination or evidence collection. **A pediatric clinician needs to further specify that while a clinician is mandated to report suspected child sexual abuse or assault of children under the age of 18 years, this mandate does not obligate the family to share information with law enforcement.**

2.5 Diagnostic Testing and Treatment of Sexually Transmitted Infections

Screening for sexually transmitted infections (STIs) is an important part of the treatment of children suspected to have been abused. **Confirmation of human immunodeficiency virus (HIV), gonorrhea, syphilis, chlamydia, trichomonas, herpes, and genital warts in children beyond the neonatal period must prompt serious consideration of child sexual abuse** (Table 2.5). Typically, 8.2% or less of children

Table 2.5 Sexually transmitted infections: diagnostic testing, treatment and reporting

Infections	Incubation	Symptoms	Testing	Prophylaxis and/or treatment	Sexual contact	Report suspected abuse
HIV-1, HIV-2	6 weeks to years	Mild viral illness; can be asymptomatic	4th generation enzyme immunoassay (HIV-1/ HIV-2 IgM &IgG, p 24 antigen)	Expert consultation suggested	Diagnostic[a]	Yes
Syphilis *Treponema pallidum*	Primary: 10–90 days	Primary: Painless genital or oral ulcers (chancres)	VDRL or RPR; if abnormal, *Treponema pallidum*-specific assay (e.g., FTA-ABS)[b]	Penicillin G	Diagnostic[a]	Yes
	Secondary: 3 weeks to 6 months after primary infection	Secondary: Palmar or plantar rash, moist wart-like lesions (Condylomata lata)				
	Tertiary: 10–30 years after primary infection	Tertiary: Gummatous skin and bone lesions, aortitis Neurosyphilis and ocular syphilis can occur at any stage				
Neisseria gonorrhoeae	3–7 days	Vaginal, urethral, rectal discharge; pharyngeal and rectal infections can be asymptomatic	Confirmed NAATs; Culture on selective media is preferred for pharynx, anus	Ceftriaxone	Diagnostic[a]	Yes
Chlamydia trachomatis	5–7 or more days; infection may persist for months after birth in genitalia (12– 16 months) and pharynx (28.5 months) (Bell 1992)	Mostly mild or asymptomatic; possible prolonged subclinical infection	Confirmed NAATs; Culture is preferred for pharynx, anus	Erythromycin; or Azithromycin; or doxycycline	Diagnostic[a]	Yes

(continued)

Table 2.5 (continued)

Infections	Incubation	Symptoms	Testing	Prophylaxis and/or treatment	Sexual contact	Report suspected abuse
Trichomonas vaginalis	5–28 days; may persist for up to 9 months after birth	Vaginal, urethral discharge; vaginal itching; dysuria	NAAT; or culture (Diamond's or InPouch TV media)	Metronidazole; or Tinidazole	Highly suspicious	Yes
Anogenital herpes HSV-1, HSV-2	2–12 days (if/when lesions)	Vesicles, ulcers; asymptomatic and subclinical infections occur in adults	HSV PCR; culture	Acyclovir; or Valacyclovir	HSV-2 highly suspicious HSV-1 suspicious	Yes
Anogenital warts (Condylomata acuminata) Human Papillomavirus	3 weeks to years (warts); months to years (cellular abnormalities)	Painless; may bleed or ulcerate; may interfere with urination or defecation	Clinical exam: Flat, cauliflower, or papular warts that are skin colored or hyperpigmented	Podofilox 0.5% liquid; or Imiquimod 3.75% or 5% cream; or cryotherapy; or surgical removal Vaccination	Suspicious	Maybe

[a] When perinatal transmission and rare nonsexual transmission are not unlikely

[b] Venereal Disease Research Laboratory (VDRL) or Rapid Plasma Reagin (RPR); if abnormal, a *Treponema pallidum*-specific assay (e.g., fluorescent treponemal antibody-absorption assay, FTA-ABS)

Adapted from (Hammerschlag & Guillén, 2010; Workowski & Bolan, 2015; Bell, 1992; AAP, 2015; Adams et al., 2018)

a   b

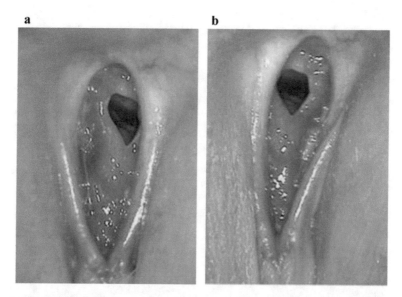

Fig. 2.34 (**a, b**) Gonorrhea vaginitis. Previously, healthy 7-year-old with new onset vaginal discharge. Culture and NAAT positive for N. gonorrhoeae. She disclosed, "[Adult male friend of father] put his private part in my private part. He said don't tell or you are going to die." Normal annular hymen noted in prone knee-chest position. Ceftriaxone administered with resolution of discharge. Diagnostic of sexual assault

aged 13 years or younger evaluated for various forms of sexual abuse or assault have one or more STIs (Girardet et al., 2009; Kelly & Koh, 2006). A subset of these children, child victims of commercial sexual exploitation, have high rates (53%) of prior STIs (Varma, Gillespie, McCracken, & Greenbaum, 2015). Children with vaginal discharge or other symptoms are more likely to have STIs (Girardet et al., 2009) (Fig. 2.34). **However, two-thirds of girls 13 years or younger with a confirmed STI have normal or nonspecific anogenital examination findings** (Girardet et al., 2009). STIs have also been documented in children with normal pharyngeal examinations (Girardet et al., 2009). Pharyngeal and anogenital cultures have been the historical gold standard for diagnosis of STIs when child sexual victimization is suspected (Kelly & Koh, 2006). Nucleic Acid Amplification Tests (NAATs) are currently being used in an increasing number of jurisdictions within the United States. This is due in part to ease of collection, compelling adult data that consistently demonstrate NAATs are more sensitive than culture, and limited but similar pediatric data (Adams et al., 2018). Use of NAATs increases detection of anogenital *Chlamydia trachomatis* and *Neisseria gonorrhoeae* in the prepubescent population (Girardet et al., 2009). In prepubescent females, the sensitivity of urine or vaginal NAATs for gonorrhea and chlamydia relative to vaginal cultures is 100% (Girardet et al., 2009). Because of the low prevalence of STIs and the medico-legal implications of STIs in the prepubescent population, the Centers for Disease Control (CDC) recommend abnormal or positive NAATs be confirmed with alternate NAATs that targets a different part of the genome (CDC, 2017).

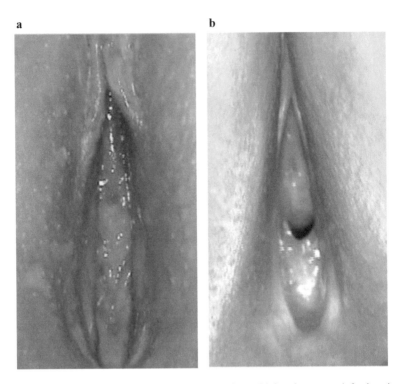

Fig. 2.35 Herpes simplex vaginitis. 8-year-old treated for multiple urinary tract infections in previous two years. No disclosure of sexual victimization. No history of oral ulcers. (**a**) Dysuria and shallow anogenital ulcers on a red base. Culture positive for HSV-1. (**b**) Normal anogenital exam with crescentic hymen noted on Day 7 of Valacyclovir treatment. Nonsexual as well as sexual transmission possible

Sexual as well as nonsexual contacts are possible modes of transmission of Herpes Simplex Virus (HSV) and Human Papillomavirus (HPV) (Adams et al., 2018; Kelly & Koh, 2006). Modes of transmissions of these potential STIs are also not mutually exclusive (Kelly & Koh, 2006). Anogenital HSV type 1 and 2 can be acquired through sexual contact, vertical transmission from mother to child, and close physical contact (e.g., diapering). Autoinoculation is a fourth possible mode of transmission for anogenital HSV (Kelly & Koh, 2006). **Children with anogenital herpes should undergo comprehensive medical and CPS evaluations in an attempt to identify the most reasonable mode(s) of transmission** (Kelly & Koh, 2006). Sexual transmission of HSV is more common in children 5 years and older, children with anogenital lesions alone, and children in which herpes simplex virus type 2 is isolated (Reading & Rannan-Eliya, 2007). **Similar to HSV, possible modes of HPV transmission in children include sexual abuse, close physical contact, autoinoculation, and/or vertical transmission.** The clinical appearance of lesions and HPV typing do not appear to be helpful in differentiating among possible modes of transmission (Fig. 2.36). There also does not appear to be consistent, readily available medical evidence about the upper age limit beyond which perinatal

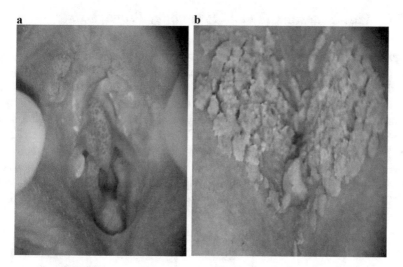

Fig. 2.36 (a, b) Condylomata acuminata (Human papillomavirus). 3-year-old with 4 months of anogenital warts that initially began on left upper thigh. Maternal anogenital warts first noted 1.5 years earlier during pregnancy with this child's younger sibling. No disclosure of abuse (limited verbal skills). Aldara® reduced bulk of lesions. No hymenal or perianal abnormalities on follow-up exam. Nonsexual as well as sexual transmission possible

transmission of HPV is not a reasonable possibility. In general, lesions appearing for the first time in 2- to 5-year-olds should prompt consideration of child sexual abuse (Hammerschlag & Guillén, 2010). The most likely mode(s) of HPV transmission may remain undetermined in a substantial minority of young children even after medical and CPS evaluations (Kelly & Koh, 2006).

The likelihood of STI transmission during child sexual abuse or assault will reflect the prevalence of a given STI in the adult population, number of perpetrators, frequency and chronicity of sexual abuse or assault, and type of sexual contact. Although the prevalence of STIs in the prepubescent population is low, STI screening is suggested when a prepubertal child:

- has experienced penetration or has evidence of recent or healed penetrative injury to the genitals, anus, or oropharynx,
- has been abused by a stranger,
- has been abused by a perpetrator known to be infected with an STI or at high risk for STIs (e.g., intravenous drug abusers, men who have sex with men, persons with multiple sexual partners, and/or a history of STIs),
- has a sibling, another relative, or another person in the household with an STI;
- lives in an area with a high rate of STIs in the community,
- has signs or symptoms of STIs (e.g., vaginal discharge or pain, genital itching or odor, urinary symptoms, and genital lesions or ulcers),
- has already been diagnosed with one STI,
- requests STI testing. (Jenny & Crawford-Jakubiak, 2013; Workowski & Bolan, 2015).

2.5.1   Post-Exposure STI and Pregnancy Prophylaxis

Prophylactic antibiotics after potential exposure to gonorrhea, chlamydia, and trichomonas are recommended for teens following acute sexual victimization that has the potential for transfer of biologic fluids. In addition to STI post-exposure prophylaxis for teens, there needs to be consideration and discussion of post-exposure pregnancy prophylaxis. Levonorgestrel (Plan B One-Step®, Levonelle® One Step, Levonelle® 1500, Isteranda®, and Upostelle®) is effective for up to 72 h (3 days) after unprotected sexual contact. Ulipristal acetate (ellaOne®) is effective for up to 120 h (5 days) (Glasier et al., 2010). Pregnancy is the only absolute contraindication for post-exposure pregnancy prophylaxis. **Because of relatively low rates of STIs among prepubescent victims, prophylactic antibiotics are not routinely**

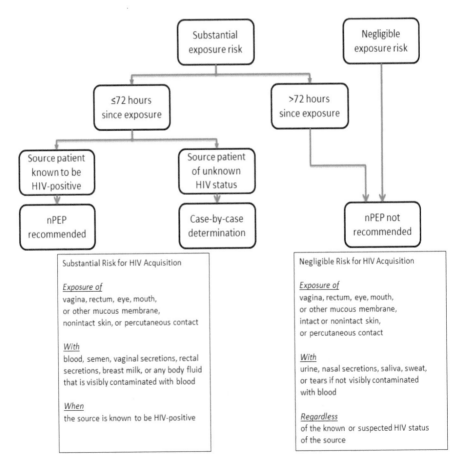

Fig. 2.37 Algorithm for evaluation and treatment of possible nonoccupational HIV exposures (Reprinted from "Sexually Transmitted Diseases Treatment Guidelines, 2015," by K. Workowski & G. Bolan, 2015, MMWR Recommendations and Reports Vol 64(3), p 107)

recommended. **Treatment of prepubescent victims for bacterial STIs is typically recommended only after confirmation of abnormal test results.** Up-to-date STI testing and treatment regimens for US-based patients are offered by the American Academy of Pediatrics and the U.S. Centers for Disease Control (Workowski & Bolan, 2015) (Table 2.5).

In children of every age, the decision about whether to initiate HIV post-exposure prophylaxis (PEP) must be made as soon as possible after an acute episode of sexual victimization that presents a substantial risk for HIV acquisition (Fig. 2.37). A local specialist in HIV treatment should be consulted when possible. The CDC also suggests the National Clinician's Post Exposure Prophylaxis Hotline, 1–888–448–4911, as a clinical resource. HIV PEP is not generally recommended when more than 72 h has elapsed since sexual victimization. It is not recommended when the victim is HIV-positive. Relevant information on HIV is also available from https://aidsinfo.nih.gov (U.S. Department of Health and Human Services, 2020).

2.6 Summary

The medical and/or forensic evaluation of the pediatric victim of sexual violence is complex. Steps include consent and counseling (on examination process, patient rights, clinician responsibilities, importance of mental health care), careful medical history taking, physical and anogenital examination(s), consideration of differential diagnoses, diagnostic testing and/or collection of forensic evidence, treatment of injury or disease, consideration of post-exposure prophylaxis, and mandated reporting (based on professional practice guidelines and jurisdictional policies). Fortunately, listening to a patient is a fundamental diagnostic skill. Careful listening and history taking will inform each additional step of the diagnostic process.

References

Adams, J., Botash, A., & Kellogg, N. (2004). Differences in hymenal morphology between adolescent girls with and without a history of consensual sexual intercourse. *Archives of Pediatrics & Adolescent Medicine, 158*(3), 280–285. https://doi.org/10.1001/archpedi.158.3.280.

Adams, J., Farst, K., & Kellogg, N. (2018). Interpretation of medical findings in suspected child sexual abuse: An update for 2018. *Journal of Pediatric and Adolescent Gynecology, 31*(3), 225–231. https://doi.org/10.1016/j.jpag.2017.12.011.

Adams, J., Harper, K., Knudson, S., & Revilla, J. (1994). Examination findings in legally confirmed child sexual abuse: It's normal to be normal. *Pediatrics, 94*(3), 310–317.

Al-Jilaihawi, S., Borg, K., Jamieson, K., Maguire, S., & Hodes, D. (2017). Clinical characteristics of children presenting with a suspicion or allegation of historic sexual abuse. *Archives of Disease in Childhood, 103*(6), 533–539. https://doi.org/10.1136/archdischild-2017-313676.

American Academy of Pediatrics (AAP). (2015). Sexually transmitted infections in adolescents and children. In D. W. Kimberlin, M. T. Brady, M. A. Jackson, & S. S. Long (Eds.), *Red book:*

2015 report of the committee on infectious diseases (30th ed., pp. 177–188). Elk Grove Village, IL: American Academy of Pediatrics. Retrieved from https://redbook.solutions.aap.org/chapter.aspx?sectionid=189640013&bookid=2205.

Anderst, J., Kellogg, N., & Jung, I. (2009). Reports of repetitive penile-genital penetration often have no definitive evidence of penetration. *Pediatrics, 124*(3), e403–e409. https://doi.org/10.1542/peds.2008-3053.

Bell, T. (1992). Chronic chlamydia trachomatis infections in infants. *JAMA: The Journal of the American Medical Association, 267*(3), 400–402. https://doi.org/10.1001/jama.267.3.400.

Berenson, A. (1995). A longitudinal study of hymenal morphology in the first 3 years of life. *Pediatrics, 95*(4), 490–496.

Berenson, A., Chacko, M., Wiemann, C., Mishaw, C., Friedrich, W., & Grady, J. (2000). A case-control study of anatomic changes resulting from sexual abuse. *American Journal of Obstetrics and Gynecology, 182*(4), 820–834. https://doi.org/10.1016/s0002-9378(00)70331-0.

Berkoff, M., Zolotor, A., Makoroff, K., Thackeray, J., Shapiro, R., & Runyan, D. (2008). Has this prepubertal girl been sexually abused? *JAMA, 300*(23), 2779–2792. https://doi.org/10.1001/jama.2008.827.

Boos, S., Rosas, A., Boyle, C., & McCann, J. (2003). Anogenital injuries in child pedestrians run over by low-speed motor vehicles: Four cases with findings that mimic child sexual abuse. *Pediatrics, 112*(1), e77–e84. https://doi.org/10.1542/peds.112.1.e77.

Botash, A., & Jean-Louis, F. (2001). Imperforate hymen: Congenital or acquired from sexual abuse? *Pediatrics, 108*(3), e53–e53. https://doi.org/10.1542/peds.108.3.e53.

Brayley-Morris, H., Sorrell, A., Revoir, A., Meakin, G., Court, D., & Morgan, R. (2015). Persistence of DNA from laundered semen stains: Implications for child sex trafficking cases. *Forensic Science International: Genetics, 19*, 165–171. https://doi.org/10.1016/j.fsigen.2015.07.016.

Christian, C., Lavelle, J., De Jong, A., Loiselle, J., Brenner, L., & Joffe, M. (2000). Forensic evidence findings in prepubertal victims of sexual assault. *Pediatrics, 106*(1), 100–104. https://doi.org/10.1542/peds.106.1.100.

Coohey, C., & O'Leary, P. (2008). Mothers' protection of their children after discovering they have been sexually abused: An information-processing perspective. *Child Abuse & Neglect, 32*(2), 245–259. https://doi.org/10.1016/j.chiabu.2007.06.002.

Drach, K., Wientzen, J., & Ricci, L. (2001). The diagnostic utility of sexual behavior problems in diagnosing sexual abuse in a forensic child abuse evaluation clinic. *Child Abuse & Neglect, 25*(4), 489–503. https://doi.org/10.1016/s0145-2134(01)00222-8.

Everson, M., & Boat, B. (1989). False allegations of sexual abuse by children and adolescents. *Journal of the American Academy of Child & Adolescent Psychiatry, 28*(2), 230–235. https://doi.org/10.1097/00004583-198903000-00014.

Friedrich, W., Fisher, J., Dittner, C., Acton, R., Berliner, L., Butler, J., … Wright, J. (2001). Child sexual behavior inventory: Normative, psychiatric, and sexual abuse comparisons. *Child Maltreatment, 6*(1), 37–49. https://doi.org/10.1177/1077559501006001004.

Gallion, H., Milam, L., & Littrell, L. (2016). Genital findings in cases of child sexual abuse: Genital vs vaginal penetration. *Journal of Pediatric and Adolescent Gynecology, 29*(6), 604–611. https://doi.org/10.1016/j.jpag.2016.05.001.

Girardet, R., Bolton, K., Lahoti, S., Mowbray, H., Giardino, A., Isaac, R., … Paes, N. (2011). Collection of forensic evidence from pediatric victims of sexual assault. *Pediatrics, 128*(2), 233–238. https://doi.org/10.1542/peds.2010-3037.

Girardet, R., Lahoti, S., Howard, L., Fajman, N., Sawyer, M., Driebe, E., … Black, C. (2009). Epidemiology of sexually transmitted infections in suspected child victims of sexual assault. *Pediatrics, 124*(1), 79–86. https://doi.org/10.1542/peds.2008-2947.

Glasier, A., Cameron, S., Fine, P., Logan, S., Casale, W., Van Horn, J., … Gainer, E. (2010). Ulipristal acetate versus levonorgestrel for emergency contraception: A randomised non-inferiority trial and meta-analysis. *The Lancet, 375*(9714), 555–562. https://doi.org/10.1016/s0140-6736(10)60101-8.

Greenbaum, V. J., Dodd, M., & McCracken, C. (2018). A short screening tool to identify victims of child sex trafficking in the health care setting. *Pediatric Emergency Care, 34*(1), 33–37. https://doi.org/10.1097/pec.0000000000000602.

Hammerschlag, M., & Guillén, C. (2010). Medical and legal implications of testing for sexually transmitted infections in children. *Clinical Microbiology Reviews, 23*(3), 493–506. https://doi.org/10.1128/cmr.00024-09.

Hébert, M., Tourigny, M., Cyr, M., McDuff, P., & Joly, J. (2009). Prevalence of childhood sexual abuse and timing of disclosure in a representative sample of adults from Quebec. *The Canadian Journal of Psychiatry, 54*(9), 631–636. https://doi.org/10.1177/070674370905400908.

Heger, A., Ticson, L., Guerra, L., Lister, J., Zaragoza, T., McConnell, G., & Morahan, M. (2002a). Appearance of the genitalia in girls selected for nonabuse. *Journal of Pediatric and Adolescent Gynecology, 15*(1), 27–35. https://doi.org/10.1016/s1083-3188(01)00136-X.

Heger, A., Ticson, L., Velasquez, O., & Bernier, R. (2002b). Children referred for possible sexual abuse: Medical findings in 2384 children. *Child Abuse & Neglect, 26*(6–7), 645–659. https://doi.org/10.1016/s0145-2134(02)00339-3.

Heppenstall-Heger, A., McConnell, G., Ticson, L., Guerra, L., Lister, J., & Zaragoza, T. (2003). Healing patterns in anogenital injuries: A longitudinal study of injuries associated with sexual abuse, accidental injuries, or genital surgery in the preadolescent child. *Pediatrics, 112*(4), 829–837. https://doi.org/10.1542/peds.112.4.829.

Hornor, G. (2010). Child sexual abuse: Consequences and implications. *Journal of Pediatric Health Care, 24*(6), 358–364. https://doi.org/10.1016/j.pedhc.2009.07.003.

Ingemann-Hansen, O., Brink, O., Sabroe, S., Sørensen, V., & Charles, A. V. (2008). Legal aspects of sexual violence—Does forensic evidence make a difference? *Forensic Science International, 180*(2–3), 98–104. https://doi.org/10.1016/j.forsciint.2008.07.009.

Iqbal, C., Jrebi, N., Zielinski, M., Benavente-Chenhalls, L., Cullinane, D., Zietlow, S., … Ishitani, M. (2010). Patterns of accidental genital trauma in young girls and indications for operative management. *Journal of Pediatric Surgery, 45*(5), 930–933. https://doi.org/10.1016/j.jpedsurg.2010.02.024.

Jenny, C. (Ed.). (2011). *Child abuse and neglect: Diagnosis, treatment, and evidence.* St. Louis, MO: Saunders/Elsevier.

Jenny, C., & Crawford-Jakubiak, J. (2013). The evaluation of children in the primary care setting when sexual abuse is suspected. *Pediatrics, 132*(2), e558–e567. https://doi.org/10.1542/peds.2013-1741.

Jenny, C., Kuhns, M., & Arakawa, F. (1987). Hymens in newborn female infants. *Pediatrics, 80*(3), 399–400.

Kellogg, N., & Parra, J. (1991). Linea vestibularis: A previously undescribed normal genital structure in female neonates. *Pediatrics, 87*(6), 926–929.

Kelly, P., & Koh, J. (2006). Sexually transmitted infections in alleged sexual abuse of children and adolescents. *Journal of Paediatrics and Child Health, 42*(7–8), 434–440. https://doi.org/10.1111/j.1440-1754.2006.00893.x.

Kogan, S. M. (2004). Disclosing unwanted sexual experiences: Results from a national sample of adolescent women. *Child Abuse & Neglect, 28*(2), 147–165. https://doi.org/10.1016/j.chiabu.2003.09.014.

Marks, S., Lamb, R., & Tzioumi, D. (2009). Do no more harm: The psychological stress of the medical examination for alleged child sexual abuse. *Journal of Paediatrics and Child Health, 45*(3), 125–132. https://doi.org/10.1111/j.1440-1754.2008.01443.x.

McCann, J., Miyamoto, S., Boyle, C., & Rogers, K. (2007a). Healing of hymenal injuries in prepubertal and adolescent girls: A descriptive study. *Pediatrics, 119*(5), e1094–e1106. https://doi.org/10.1542/peds.2006-0964.

McCann, J., Miyamoto, S., Boyle, C., & Rogers, K. (2007b). Healing of nonhymenal genital injuries in prepubertal and adolescent girls: A descriptive study. *Pediatrics, 120*(5), 1000–1011. https://doi.org/10.1542/peds.2006-0230.

McCann, J., & Voris, J. (1993). Perianal injuries resulting from sexual abuse: A longitudinal study. *Pediatrics, 91*, 390–397.

McCann, J., Voris, J., & Simon, M. (1992). Genital injuries resulting from sexual abuse: A longitudinal study. *Pediatrics, 89*(2), 307–317.

McCann, J., Voris, J., Simon, M., & Wells, R. (1989). Perianal findings in prepubertal children selected for nonabuse: A descriptive study. *Child Abuse & Neglect, 13*(2), 179–193. https://doi.org/10.1016/0145-2134(89)90005-7.

Myhre, A., Adams, J., Kaufhold, M., Davis, J., Suresh, P., & Kuelbs, C. (2013). Anal findings in children with and without probable anal penetration: A retrospective study of 1115 children referred for suspected sexual abuse. *Child Abuse & Neglect, 37*(7), 465–474. https://doi.org/10.1016/j.chiabu.2013.03.011.

Myhre, A., Berntzen, K., & Bratlid, D. (2003). Genital anatomy in non-abused preschool girls. *Acta Paediatrica, 92*(12), 1453–1462.

Palusci, V., Cox, E., Shatz, E., & Schultze, J. (2006). Urgent medical assessment after child sexual abuse. *Child Abuse & Neglect, 30*(4), 367–380. https://doi.org/10.1016/j.chiabu.2005.11.002.

Peterson, M., Holbrook, J., Von Hales, D., Smith, N. L., & Staker, L. (1992). Contributions of the history, physical examination, and laboratory investigation in making medical diagnoses. *Obstetrical & Gynecological Survey, 47*(10), 711–712.

Reading, R., & Rannan-Eliya, Y. (2007). Evidence for sexual transmission of genital herpes in children. *Archives of Disease in Childhood, 92*(7), 608–613. https://doi.org/10.1136/adc.2005.086835.

Schaeffer, P., Leventhal, J., & Asnes, A. (2011). Children's disclosures of sexual abuse: Learning from direct inquiry. *Child Abuse & Neglect, 35*(5), 343–352. https://doi.org/10.1016/j.chiabu.2011.01.014.

Sjöberg, R. L., & Lindblad, F. (2002). Limited disclosure of sexual abuse in children whose experiences were documented by videotape. *The American Journal of Psychiatry, 159*(2), 312–314. https://doi.org/10.1176/appi.ajp.159.2.312.

Starling, S., & Jenny, C. (1997). Forensic examination of adolescent female genitalia: The Foley catheter technique. *Archives of Pediatrics & Adolescent Medicine, 151*(1), 102–103. https://doi.org/10.1001/archpedi.1997.02170380106020.

Survivors' Bill of Rights Act of 2016, Pub. L. No. 114–236. (2016). Retrieved from https://www.congress.gov/bill/114th-congress/house-bill/5578

Thackeray, J., Hornor, G., Benzinger, E., & Scribano, P. (2011). Forensic evidence collection and DNA identification in acute child sexual assault. *Pediatrics, 128*(2), 227–232. https://doi.org/10.1542/peds.2010-3498.

U.S. Department of Health and Human Services. (2020). AIDSinfo. Retrieved from aidsinfo.nih.gov

Varma, S., Gillespie, S., McCracken, C., & Greenbaum, V. (2015). Characteristics of child commercial sexual exploitation and sex trafficking victims presenting for medical care in the United States. *Child Abuse & Neglect, 44*, 98–105. https://doi.org/10.1016/j.chiabu.2015.04.004.

Violence Against Women Reauthorization Act of 2013, Pub. L. No. 113–4. (2013). Retrieved from https://www.congress.gov/bill/113th-congress/senate-bill/47

Watkeys, J., Price, L., Upton, P., & Maddocks, A. (2008). The timing of medical examination following an allegation of sexual abuse: Is this an emergency? *Archives of Disease in Childhood, 93*(10), 851–856. https://doi.org/10.1136/adc.2007.123604.

Workowski, K., & Bolan, G. (2015). Sexually transmitted diseases treatment guidelines, 2015. *Centers for Disease Control and Prevention MMWR Recomm Rep, 64*(3). https://www.cdc.gov/std/tg2015/tg-2015-print.pdf.

Chapter 3
Related Issues

In this chapter, a number of issues are addressed related to the healthcare approach to child sexual abuse. First, the issues related to the timing of a victim's disclosure of child sexual abuse are explored. Next, the accuracy of the disclosure is considered since the truthfulness of a child's disclosure or outcry related to the abuse as relayed to the healthcare provider during the evaluation may be questioned during the law enforcement aspects of the investigation. Next, the evolving literature surrounding the risk of maltreatment for children with disabilities is reviewed. Additionally, the emerging concern about the risk for child maltreatment that may arise from participation with a variety of youth-serving organizations is reviewed. The risk posed by the Internet specifically related to online sexual solicitation is addressed. Finally, the reality of the backlash against child sexual abuse victims is considered as well.

3.1   Delayed Disclosures in Child Sexual Abuse

Paige A. Culotta

It is estimated that 1 in 8 children worldwide are sexually abused though this is thought to be an underestimation as victimization is underreported (Collin-Vezina, De La Sablonniere-Griffin, Palmer, & Milne, 2015; Kellogg and the Committee on Child Abuse and Neglect, 2005. Disclosure is the most important aspect in discovery of child sexual abuse as corroborating evidence is rare (Goodman-Brown, Edelstein, Goodman, Jones, & Gordon, 2003; Heger, Ticson, Velasquez, & Bernier, 2002). A common question after a child reveals that they have been a victim of sexual abuse is why now? Why wait months, years to divulge this information? While one may expect children to seek an adult's help immediately to stop this abuse, the reality is that between 55 and 70% of victims have a delay in disclosure of sexual abuse until after adulthood (Alaggia, 2010; London, Bruck, Wright, &

© The Author(s) 2020
T. S. Hinds, A. P. Giardino, *Child Sexual Abuse*, SpringerBriefs in Public
Health, https://doi.org/10.1007/978-3-030-52549-1_3

Ceci, 2008). Even in instances where evidence is available, many children deny the abuse (Malloy, Lyon, & Quas, 2007). Countless factors including culture, family circumstances, social concerns, shame, self-blame, fear of consequences, expectations of negative reactions, and relationship to the offender, contribute to a child's willingness to reach out to an adult for help (Goodman-Brown et al., 2003).

Abuse is not always recognized as such. Over 90% of perpetrators have been shown to be known to a child, many of those being family members and father figures (Crisma, Bascelli, Paci, & Romito, 2004). Children in these difficult situations, especially when there is a close relationship with the perpetrator, have often undergone a period of grooming which progresses over time (Berlinger & Conte, 1990; Goodman-Brown et al., 2003; Jackson, Newall, & Backett-Milburn, 2015). This may begin as seemingly innocent contact, gaining a child's trust (Berlinger & Conte, 1990; Kellogg and the Committee on Child Abuse and Neglect, 2005). Manipulation by the abuser sends a message that this behavior is "ok" or "normal," that there is a "special relationship," that they are chosen or favored over others (Berlinger & Conte, 1990; Jackson et al., 2015). Abusers may make promises that it will "never happen again" and or attempt to justify their actions (Berlinger & Conte, 1990; Jackson et al., 2015). In addition to manipulation, abusers often use the power dynamic to instill fear in their victims, threatening harm or violence to the child themselves or their loved ones (Craven, Brown, & Gilchrist, 2006).

Research shows that a majority of perpetrators are known to the child and thus the relationship to the abuser is often highly complex (Berlinger & Conte, 1995; Heger et al., 2002). A child may be fearful of violence from this abuser but also have a sense of closeness or loyalty, with concern about what would happen to that person if the abuse is discovered (Mian, Wehrspan, Klajner-Diamond, LeBaron, & Winder, 1986; Reitsema & Grietens, 2016). In studies, children frequently expressed not only a fear of consequences for themselves but also for their abuser: being arrested, having to leave the home, etc. (Jensen, Gulbrandsen, Mossige, Reichelt, & Thersland, 2005). As expected, with this bond, disclosure is delayed more often in cases where the abuser is within the child's family (Kogan, 2004).

Relation of age to time of disclosure varies and is often dependent on the type of abuse and the age of onset, earlier resulting in an increase in delay (Kogan, 2004). Studies have shown that younger children are less likely to disclose intrafamilial abuse, while adolescents are more likely to delay disclosure when the offender is someone outside of the family (Hershkowitz, Lanes, & Lamb, 2007; Leach, Powell, Sharman, & Anglim, 2017; London et al., 2008). Developmental barriers also play a role. Young children may lack the cognitive ability to understand that what is happening is wrong and experience further confusion about the abuse (Allnock & Miller, 2013; Collin-Vezina et al., 2015; Hershkowitz et al., 2007; London, Bruck, Ceci, & Shuman, 2005). Moreover, they lack the vocabulary to explain the behavior or situation and their indirect attempts go unnoticed (Allnock & Miller, 2013; Collin-Vezina et al., 2015). This can be compounded by societal factors including the absence of discussion about sexuality even in mainstream education, resulting in children being unaware of what is normal, and what is inappropriate or abuse (Collin-Vezina et al., 2015). Older children's awareness of these social taboos can influence secrecy as can their recognition of the impact telling will have (Collin-Vezina et al., 2015).

Feelings of shame, embarrassment, self-blame, and guilt are commonly identified by victims as contributing to a delay in disclosure (Collin-Vezina et al., 2015; Hamilton, Brubacher, & Powell, 2016; Hunter, 2011). These feelings vary based on the child's gender and cultural and religious beliefs. Shame is commonly reported by victims and is exacerbated in many social settings with inadequate teaching, forbidden words, and the taboo of the discussion of sexuality (Fontes & Plummer, 2010; Hershkowitz et al., 2007; McElvaney, Greene, & Hogan, 2012). Female victims were more likely to identify self-blame and guilt for causing or failing to stop abuse (Goodman-Brown et al., 2003; Jackson et al., 2015). Certain sexual scripts relay that men are unable to control themselves and it is the woman's job to prevent this aggression with her behavior or clothing (Fontes & Plummer, 2010). In families with traditional roles—a dominant, powerful father and submissive mother—victims were less likely to discuss their abuse due to difficulty battling against the expectation that children should "be seen but not heard" (Alaggia, 2010; Alaggia & Kirshenbaum, 2005).

While not consistent in all studies, it is generally suggested that male victims are more hesitant to disclose (Finkelhor, 1990; Goodman-Brown et al., 2003). Boys often fear stigmatization (Alaggia, 2010; Fontes & Plummer, 2010). Male victims may question their own sexuality and fear being labeled homosexual when the offender is also male (Alaggia, 2010; Collin-Vezina et al., 2015; Fontes & Plummer, 2010). Societal roles often stress masculinity and strength, leaving male victims to feel inadequacy in being unable to prevent the abuse, or even ridiculed for not enjoying the sexual act (Alaggia, 2010; Collin-Vezina et al., 2015; Fontes & Plummer, 2010). Abusers will use these feelings to their advantage, telling their victims that they will get in trouble if actions are found out, or that the child is at fault because they did not say no (Berlinger & Conte, 1990; Goodman-Brown et al., 2003). In addition to physical intimidation, victims are threatened with abandonment or rejection (Berlinger & Conte, 1990; Goodman-Brown et al., 2003). Households where a child experiences poly-victimization, low levels of family support, and a general feeling of insecurity in the home have a significantly decreased likelihood that a disclosure would be made (Collin-Vezina et al., 2015; Hershkowitz et al., 2007; Malloy et al., 2007; Tashjian, Goldfarb, Goodman, Quas, & Edelstein, 2016). Children who are maltreated by their parents often perceive a lack of support, with negative expectations at times of difficult situations (Tashjian et al., 2016).

While the abuse itself causes a child significant distress, so does the process of disclosure which often comes at an immense cost to the child: problems for the family, loss of support, financial burden, and tarnished reputations (Fontes & Plummer, 2010). In over 20 years of research, it has remained constant that fear of a family crisis causes monumental concern to a child and influences their decision to keep abuse secret even more than physical threats of violence (Hunter, 2011). All adults in a study by Hunter et al. reported disclosure-related trauma, especially when the traumatic event occurred in childhood (Hunter, 2011; Ullman, 2007). A child struggles with many aspects of this endeavor as described in three phases: active withholding, conflict between the desire to disclose and wish to keep this secret, and finally, selective disclosure (McElvaney et al., 2012).

In active withholding, a child consciously does not reveal their abuse (McElvaney et al., 2012). This is a protective mechanism, which for some is a form of denial or minimizing the abuse but for others can also be a means of developing a sense of control (McElvaney et al., 2012). He or she may then battle feelings of wanting to reveal this information while also having the desire to keep it a secret, wondering how others will react and what the consequences will be (McElvaney et al., 2012). Once the decision to disclose is made, then comes the choice of a confidant and how to communicate this information with a careful selection of timing, context, and privacy (Jensen et al., 2005; McElvaney et al., 2012). Studies have identified a barrier at this part of the journey to be a child's lack of a trusted person to turn to (Alaggia, 2010; Allnock & Miller, 2013; Tashjian et al., 2016).

Adverse family circumstances, including divorce; bereavement; or a non-offending parent with mental illness, substance use, or otherwise under significant stress, deter disclosure as the child worries that this caregiver will be unable to handle the information or take protective measures (Alaggia & Kirshenbaum, 2005; Allnock & Miller, 2013; Jackson et al., 2015; Jensen et al., 2005; Kogan, 2004). It is not appealing for a victim to conduct this conversation with a person who shows little interest or becomes distressed (Jensen et al., 2005). When a confidant is identified, a child carefully chooses an opportunity to begin this conversation, a task felt to be extremely difficult (Jensen et al., 2005). The child often seeks a private setting in which there is a connection to the subject matter, such as a television show, sexual education at school, or a situation in which a child is expected to have contact with the abuser (Jensen et al., 2005). Children and adults in retrospective studies often note a lack of opportunity to tell as a significant barrier, followed by the anticipated response by the chosen confidant, most commonly a mother or peer (Jensen et al., 2005; Malloy et al., 2007).

A disclosure is an ongoing dialogue, an interactive process, between the child and an adult that develops based on the reaction that is received (Flam & Haugstvedt, 2013; Jensen et al., 2005). The child will often give subtle clues or "test balloons" to the adults around them as a way to evaluate how this person will react to a disclosure (Flam & Haugstvedt, 2013). These first signs are often small and indirect but are used to build a context and opportunity for discussion (Flam & Haugstvedt, 2013; Jensen et al., 2005). A child may express reservation about a situation related to a certain person or question a rule as a sign of unease at a selected time connected to a trusted person (Flam & Haugstvedt, 2013; Jensen et al., 2005). He or she may ask to quit piano lessons, or state that anyone but Uncle John can babysit. This is the first opportunity for the adult to listen, open a dialogue, and begin to formulate a framework to further this discussion (Jensen et al., 2005). Minimizing, normalizing, or correcting the expression with closed questions will quickly shut down the conversation and send a message that the discussion is not supported (Flam & Haugstvedt, 2013; Jensen et al., 2005). Uncle John is so nice, he loves spending time with you; Julie is an excellent piano teacher, you are lucky to have her. While it may not be intention, children and adult victims of child sexual abuse note this lack of recognition as a reason for nondisclosure, saying, "No one asked" (Allnock & Miller, 2013).

Another roadblock to disclosure that has been studied is a child's anticipation of unsupportive reactions or disbelief of the information revealed, and this is often not inaccurate (Hershkowitz et al., 2007; Jackson et al., 2015; Jensen et al., 2005). Fear of disbelief was found to be one of the most important factors to impede disclosure (Hershkowitz et al., 2007; Jackson et al., 2015). Dismissive responses or inadequate suggestions, such as, "Always wear underwear and pants to bed at grandpa's house," sends a message to a child to keep quiet (Fontes & Plummer, 2010). Children are astute and often accurately interpret the way their disclosure will be received (Hershkowitz et al., 2007; Jensen et al., 2005; Reitsema & Grietens, 2016). With mothers being the most common person young people disclose to, less than 50% both believe and take protective measures for their child (Jackson et al., 2015; Pintello & Zuravin, 2001). Caregivers were less likely to believe and take appropriate action when they were in a sexual relationship with the accused or when the relationship is dependent (Jensen et al., 2005; Reitsema & Grietens, 2016). Additionally, if the child had exhibited sexualized behaviors, mothers were less likely to be supportive of the disclosure (Pintello & Zuravin, 2001). Studies show that negative responses to disclosure have profound psychological effects, including post-traumatic stress disorder, regardless of when the disclosure is made (Ullman, 2007). Additionally, victims are more likely to recant in situations where the response has not been supportive (Malloy et al., 2007).

An overwhelming majority of abuse is intrafamilial, a factor that is not surprisingly significant in contributing to nondisclosure and stress within a family (Bicanic, Hehenkamp, van de Putte, van Wijk, & de Jongh, 2015; Goodman-Brown et al., 2003). Children fear that remaining in the current situation after disclosure may be unbearable, putting them or their loved ones at increased risk for retaliation and escalation in the abuse, or worse, they would be ostracized from the family themselves (Fontes & Plummer, 2010). The converse concern is that if they are believed, they will be responsible for disrupting the family structurally and, in many cases, financially when the abuser is the provider.

With the vast hurdles a victim of child sexual abuse must overcome prior to disclosure, certain items are recognized to promote reporting. Studies find that when a person recognizes and asks about a child's struggle, he or she is more likely to make a disclosure (Allnock & Miller, 2013). Escalating violence and being unable to continue coping with the abuse can trigger a spontaneous disclosure though the intent of disclosure is not always to stop abuse but is in many cases to protect others and gain support (Allnock & Miller, 2013). While the disclosure of abuse is particularly distressing, the experience is noted to be positive in settings where a child felt they were believed, received emotional support, and some action of protection was taken (Allnock & Miller, 2013). These items are not only important to ensuring abuse stops but also reflecting positively on a child's psychological prognosis (Bicanic et al., 2015; Hamilton et al., 2016).

Sexual abuse is both physically and emotionally devastating to the child victim, and it is worsened by the child's internal battle of how to manage this secret. The only way to ensure abuse is stopped and the offender is prevented from continuing on this destructive path is when it is revealed by the child victim. While reasons for delay are multifactorial, they significantly impact the child involved. Those in the field of child protection must take this information and provide education that will enable adults to recognize the emotional intelligence of a child, remain sensitive to clues of their discomfort, and continue open communication with active listening and support to encourage a child that they can reach out and will be protected.

3.2 Accuracy of History/Interview in Child Sexual Abuse

Marcella M. Donaruma-Kwoh

A clear and consistent disclosure from a child who has been sexually abused is the cornerstone to successfully connecting that child and family with appropriate medical, mental health, and investigative resources as well as eventually prosecuting the abuser. Physical signs of sexual abuse are rarely present. In a 2002 pediatric sexual abuse study of 1652 children who disclosed abuse, only 4.4% had an abnormal examination, even though 68.6% of the 1652 children had disclosed anal or vaginal penetration (Heger et al., 2002). Therefore, even in cases in which the child victims report penetrative abuse, the exam is most likely to show normal anogenital anatomy, emphasizing the critical role of the child's history in the evaluation of these patients.

The pediatric medical literature is sparse on the assessment of child sexual abuse histories; rather, the lion's share of the data stems from journals for professionals in mental health or legal fora. Thus, it is unsurprising that the reliability and veracity of a child's disclosure for the prosecution figures largely in those publications. A recent literature search demonstrated that between 2 and 8% of reports of child sexual abuse were viewed as false by the various professionals involved in the child's evaluation. Blatantly false reports were found to be motivated by revenge, mental illness, and less commonly, by adolescents hoping to avoid getting in trouble (Block, Foster, Pierce, Berkoff, & Runyan, 2013). It is important to note that the validity of the "false" categorization of a given child's disclosure cannot be determined. The extent and content of a child's disclosure is influenced by a myriad of factors, so the purpose of this section is to explore interpretation of validity of a disclosure based on the child, the child's caregiver, and society's response to a disclosure.

3.2.1 The Child

One of the first things a pediatrician is taught in training is "children are not just little adults." This mantra also holds true for child disclosure of sexual abuse. A child's experience of disclosure is influenced by age, developmental stage, upbringing, environment, and their knowledge of their own body. Eliciting and interpreting a child's outcry the same way one would an adult's history has the potential to lead to confusion and misinterpretation.

Age is a well-studied factor influencing disclosure. Multiple studies, including the Heger sexual abuse study in 2002, found a positive association between age and likelihood of disclosure (Heger et al., 2002). The Heger study found that in the 2384 children referred for evaluation, the group that disclosed abuse was statistically older than the group that had not disclosed abuse; on average, children who disclosed were 7.8 years old, versus 4.5 years in the nondisclosing group (Heger et al., 2002). Another study of 527 children between 3 and 16 years found that likelihood of disclosure increased until 11 years, then decreased (Leach et al., 2017). Overall, these and other studies initially found that younger children are less likely to disclose than older children (Hershkowitz, Horowitz, & Lamb, 2005; Leclerc & Wortley, 2015; Lippert, Cross, Jones, & Walsh, 2009).

3.2.1.1 Before School Age Children (0–5 Years)

Researchers have shown that young children (<7 years in most studies) may not disclose because they are less likely to recognize inappropriate sexual behaviors as abuse, may not understand the purpose of a forensic interview, or may be limited in very young cases by lack of language or knowledge to describe inappropriate behaviors (Hershkowitz et al., 2005; Leach et al., 2017; Lippert et al., 2009; Steward, Bussey, Goodman, & Saywitz, 1993). In association with age, language development factors heavily into the perception of the history's validity.

The subtle landmarks of receptive/expressive language development are important when considering disclosures from very young children, especially when combined with cognitive/social skills milestones. Preschoolers (3–5 years) can speak in sentences and have vocabularies that include most familiar words. A 3-year-old can begin to understand the concepts of "in," "on," and "under" (CDC NCBDDD, 2019a), but their ability to communicate about and understand the concept of time is not yet well developed, for example, they may confuse whether something happened before or after a causal event, or they may be better at showing a sequence of events via lining up pictures than explaining it verbally (Bullock, Gelman, & Baillargeon, 1982). It is reasonable to expect children to answer "what," "where," and "who" questions by age 3, but they will not fully understand "when," "why," and "how" aspects of history-telling (Steward et al., 1993). A 4-year-old can begin to reliably and correctly use the terms "he" and "she" and understands the idea of same and different (CDC NCBDDD, 2019b). Studies have also shown that at this age most children begin to understand what a lie is and perceive that a lie is not socially acceptable. A 4-year-old child can understand the moral difference of lying with intent to deceive vs. committing an accidental misdeed (Bussey, 1992). A 5-year-old begins to understand real and make-believe and can speak in future tense (CDC NCBDDD, 2019c). These milestones are important for forming interview questions and interpreting stories told by young children.

Commonly, younger children interviewed by experienced interviewers will provide short answers to open-ended questions and tend to omit details, i.e., "lies of omission" (Hershkowitz, Lamb, Orbach, Katz, & Horowitz, 2012). However, these children can also be influenced by suggestibility (i.e., introducing false information via questioning). A systematic review of literature by Ceci and Friedman (2000) showed that children, especially young children, are susceptible to suggestion in interviewing, especially when interviewed with directed questioning (yes and no questions, forced choice questions). This means that unskilled interviewers could inadvertently introduce false information into a child's narrative during questioning due to suggestive interviewing techniques, and Binet noted that this information can persist in a child's memories during retesting (as cited in Ceci & Friedman, 2000). Some court rooms and interviewers attempt to prevent suggestion bias by having the child practice answering, "I don't know" to common questions before beginning questioning, and praising children for answering, "I don't know" (Ahern, Stolzenberg, & Lyon, 2015).

3.2.1.2 School Age Children and Adolescents (6–11 Years)

As children enter school and later enter puberty, they begin to understand more complex social relationships and social structures. They care about other people liking them and perceive their role in their environment (CDC NCBDDD, 2019d, 2019e). By first grade, most children provide accurate recall of past events (Steward et al., 1993). These children are typically able to provide implicit (fear, shame) and explicit (reflecting on why they were abused) reflections about their abuse events, as well as the details of contact, associations with pain, and descriptions of abuser coercion or threats (Hassan, Hotz, Killion, & Vicken, 2015). After age 10, most children are likely to provide fuller disclosures with more accurate details about the timing associated with events (Orbach & Lamb, 2007).

Specific data on factors influencing disclosure in this age group is limited. One study found that school age children had higher rates of reporting intrafamilial abuse than young children (postulated to be due to less reliance on caregiver) as well as the highest rate of reporting extrafamilial abuse. This was thought to be due to two factors: school age children can recognize abusive behaviors as abnormal treatment, unlike young children, and are less likely to perceive a "relationship" with the abuser, unlike adolescent victims. (Leach et al., 2017). The same study also found increased disclosure after 12 months (late disclosure) in the school age group, suggested to be related to fear of consequences from disclosing and greater feelings of responsibility for the abuse (Goodman-Brown et al., 2003; Leach et al., 2017; Malloy, Brubacher, & Lamb, 2011). Children in this age group have also been reported to "lie" about their abuse but by denying or minimizing the events that have occurred rather than inventing an abusive narrative (Sjöberg & Lindblad, 2002).

3.2.1.3   Adolescents (12–18 Years)

Adolescents represent a unique age group in child sexual abuse because these children are progressing into adulthood and may have begun having their own dating or sexual relationships. At this stage, children often have complex relationships with their caregivers as they become more independent and seek to be given more responsibility and freedom from the traditional dependent child/caregiver relationship. Children in this age group are almost equally as likely to disclose their sexual abuse history to a peer as they are a trusted adult (Kogan, 2004; Schaeffer, Leventhal, & Gottsegen Asnes, 2011). A UK survey-based study of public opinion showed that in general, adults perceive older children to be less credible than younger children when making similar disclosures of sexual abuse (Davies & Rogers, 2009). This type of bias can create difficulty in formulating the appropriate response to an abuse outcry, from the family unit to investigative agencies, or with jury members. Another unique aspect of adolescent outcries is that as age increases, the likelihood of a victim deciding to not pursue charges increases because in most cases the offender was a "boyfriend" or "girlfriend" (Bunting, 2008). Though the literature varies, some studies have found that the reporting of sexual abuse declines in adolescence (Leach et al., 2017), theorized to be related to these boyfriend/girlfriend relationships with abusers, fear of retaliation, or self-blame (Goodman-Brown et al., 2003; Hershkowitz et al., 2005; Malloy et al., 2011). Older children also may be more likely to provide a tentative disclosure, which is a disclosure characterized by a lack of certainty or clarity, such as repetitions of "I don't know" or "I can't remember" or attempts to deflect the course of the conversation; younger children are less likely to do so. Interestingly, the type of sexual abuse a child had suffered was not linked to increased likelihood of tentative disclosure, but an adult perpetrator and unsupportive family members were both associated with tentative disclosures (Anderson, 2016).

3.2.2   The Caregiver

The response of a caregiver to a child's outcry of sexual abuse can be belief, disbelief, uncertainty, or indifference, with a host of overlying emotional responses. Caregiver support of child sexual abuse survivors can shape an adaptive response to that life stress; this support may be impaired as non-offending parents are thrust into the role of navigating potential economic and social challenges in addition to the psychological burden of identifying the occurrence of their child's abuse. Parents of sexually abused children self-report an increase in inconsistent parenting, which can in turn impact their child's ability to develop resilience to current and future life stressors (Jobe-Shields, Swiecicki, Fritz, Stinnette, & Hanson, 2016).

Malloy showed that in a study involving 58 children who recanted a substantiated disclosure of sexual abuse, children with disbelieving family member were more likely to recant the claim of sexual abuse (Malloy, Mugno, Rivard, Lyon, & Quas, 2016). Family members who believed and supported the claim of sexual abuse were found to be protective against recantation (Malloy et al., 2016). Another study found that, on average, children supported by their mothers had a shorter latency to disclosure of sexual abuse (0.75 years) (Rakovec-Felser & Vidovic, 2016). This study also showed that a mother showing ambivalence to a claim of sexual abuse lengthened the delay to disclosure even further than disbelief (mean 6.93 years vs. mean 3.65 years) (Rakovec-Felser & Vidovic, 2016). Parental disbelief at time of disclosure was also found to be related to self-blame in the child (Melville, Kellogg, Perez, & Lukefahr, 2014).

The abuse effects on the caregiver must also be emphasized. A study in South Africa found that mothers of child sexual abuse victims experienced secondary trauma from the child's abuse, including guilt, self-blame, depression, emotional pain, and suicidal ideation. Many reported isolating themselves from friends and family because of fear of blame or negative responses. Mothers also were left to cope with the financial burden of transporting the child to doctors' and legal visits, sometimes without the support of the breadwinner of the family if they were the perpetrators (Masilo & Davhana-Maselesele, 2016). A further study in New Zealand explored caregiver needs via survey following child sexual abuse. A fifth of surveyed caregivers reported physical symptoms of sleep or appetite loss following finding out about their child's sexual abuse, and an equal percentage reported not knowing how to respond to the abuse. A third of the sample reported they were doing "not well," and 10% said they were avoiding the issue of their child's abuse. When asked what they needed to do better, almost half of non-offending adults said they needed help responding to their child and 21.7% wanted therapy for themselves (van Toledo & Seymour, 2016). Caretakers of children who had suffered sexual abuse, both extrafamilial and intrafamilial, have also reported symptoms of major depressive disorder afterward and accessed mental health services, with increased prescriptions for antidepressants in the wake of their child's disclosure. Mothers and fathers of child victims also reported more psychological distress than the general population. Mothers reported more symptoms of post-traumatic stress, a finding most prominent in high income families (Cyr et al., 2016).

These studies highlight the importance of the caregiver in a child's response to sexual abuse for the child's mental health as well as for future prosecution. They also draw attention to a need for support for caregivers who are victims of secondary trauma from their child's abuser.

3.2.3 Society

Society responds to child sexual abuse in various venues. A frequent concern is the validity of the outcry, whether in the community or in the courtroom. In response, the legal system devotes resources for research to improve validity of disclosures and minimize waste. Block et al. (2013) explored the improvement of conviction rates of child sexual abuse offenders with multiple forensic interviews for children. They found that disclosure improved with repeat interviews, with an increased conviction rate of 6.1% based on the new information, and with an associated cost per child estimated around $100,000 (Block et al., 2013). The costs of convicting child sexual abuse offenders, ostensibly to protect the community's children, is an ongoing discussion.

Society also provides its own out-of-court judgment of child sexual abuse victims. A study of forensic interview videos showed that victims who were not emotional during testimony had a negative evaluation by prosecutors (Castelli & Goodman, 2014). Another study showed that sexual abuse testimony reviewed by law students was determined to be less credible if the child was reported to have ADHD or Asperger syndrome (Lainpelto, Isaksson, & Lindblad, 2016).

3.2.4 Multicultural Considerations

A newer topic that has entered the discussion is the role that race may play in a child's likelihood to disclose their abuse history. In a review of 522 forensic interviews, African American and Caucasian children demonstrated an increased tendency to disclose their abuse when "cross mixed" with an interviewer of the other race (Fisher, Mackey, Langendoen, & Barnard, 2016). Further research has looked into specific racial identities and the experience of disclosure.

3.2.4.1 China/Taiwan

Some studies have shown lower rates of child sexual abuse in China, but acknowledge the possibility of inhibited disclosure. Authors suggest this lower rate of abuse is related to Confucian values, variations in the perception of masculinity, and different family structure/values in China (Finkelhor, Ji, Mikton, & Dunne, 2013). However, a more recent review of disclosure at Taiwanese psychiatric hospitals supported that Chinese children are as equally likely to disclose sexual abuse as western counterparts (Wang, Lu, & Tsai, 2016). American studies of child sexual abuse victims typically underrepresent children of Asian extraction; clearly, this population is in need of further study.

3.2.4.2 Australian Aboriginals

Children who are part of the Australian aboriginal population can experience sexual abuse in a distinct way. Children in this group experience shame for similar reasons as western children, but they also experience shame when someone draws attention to them, when they feel singled out or selected, or when they meet strangers. Children in this population that endorses shame from sexual abuse required more prompting and reminders from interviewers to disclose (Hamilton et al., 2016).

3.2.5 Conclusion

A clear and consistent disclosure of sexual abuse can be a challenge to elicit from a pediatric patient, and more tentative disclosures may be more difficult to interpret. A child's disclosure is a nuanced aspect of the medical history both in its content and our response to it. This is in conflict with both our child protection and legal system, each of which demands a binary interpretation of information that so often presents to providers along a continuum. Our response must be guided by a reliable and thorough evaluation and an analytic thought process to create a management plan aimed at helping the child achieve their healthiest potential in mind and body.

3.3 Risk of Child Sexual Abuse of Children with Disabilities

Clinicians have long been concerned that children with disabilities may be at higher risk for child maltreatment, specifically child sexual abuse, when compared to children without special healthcare needs. A number of early clinical studies pointed to this heightened risk of child maltreatment in various clinical samples of children being treated for a variety of disabilities and medical conditions (Hudson & Giardino, 1996). Later, several increasingly rigorous epidemiologic studies provided stronger evidence for the existence of an increased risk for child maltreatment (Child Welfare Information Gateway, 2018). The finding of increased risk of maltreatment among children with special healthcare needs has not been consistent; however, the overall trend has been supportive of the initial clinical suspicion that this special group of patients may have unique circumstances that place them at risk for child maltreatment in general, and in some cases, for an increased risk of child sexual abuse (Child Welfare Information Gateway, 2018). In this section, the definition of children with special healthcare needs is provided, an overview of the literature that supports an increased risk for this population of child maltreatment will be explored, and then the emerging data that supports specific subsets of those children with special healthcare needs being at increased risk for child sexual abuse is presented.

3.3.1 Definition of Children with Disabilities

Children with disabilities describes in varying detail the range of medical, emotional, and developmental conditions that distinguish these from the routinely developing general population of children served in the typical primary care setting. In the healthcare setting, the term children with special healthcare needs may be used to describe children with disabilities as well as children with conditions that make them more medically complex. For this chapter, the designation of children with disabilities is broad enough to capture the at-risk population being addressed.

Definitions Related to Children with Disabilities

Children with Disabilities:
According to the Individuals with Disabilities Education Act, the term 'child with a disability' means a child (1) with intellectual disabilities, hearing impairments (including deafness), speech or language impairments, visual impairments (including blindness), serious emotional disturbance, orthopedic impairments, autism, traumatic brain injury, other health impairments, or specific learning disabilities and (2) who, by reason thereof, needs special education and related services (IDEA, 1990).

Children with Special Healthcare Needs:
The federal Maternal and Child Health Bureau defines children with special health care needs as those who have or are in increased risk for a chronic physical, developmental, behavioral, or emotional condition and who also require health and related services of a type or amount beyond that required by children generally. Children and youth with special health care needs and their families often need services from multiple systems—health care, public health, education, mental health, and social services (USDHHS, 2019).

Depending on the epidemiologic data used, the estimate of the number of children with a disability varies (Turchi & Giardino, 2019). Using a fairly strict definition and limiting the estimate to school age children between 5 and 17 years of age, the 2010 U.S. Census found that 5.2% of school age children have a disability (U.S. Census Bureau, 2011). However, using the more inclusive federal Maternal and Child Health Bureau definition, the National Survey of Children's Health found an overall national prevalence of 19% of children with special healthcare needs (Bethell et al., 2015). Estimates are that one in five families with children in the United States have at least one child who qualifies as having a special healthcare need (USDHHS, 2014). Therefore, children with disabilities and special healthcare needs represent a large subset of the overall child and adolescent population, which confirms the need for healthcare providers and the healthcare system to pay careful attention to their unique care needs.

The quantification of the actual increased risk of maltreatment among this population also varies. According to the U.S. Department of Health and Human Services' Children's Bureau, an accurate estimate of the rate of maltreatment among children with disabilities is difficult because of varying reporting requirements and data collection methods along with the use of different definitions among the States (Child Welfare Information Gateway, 2018). One recent estimate using 2014 data reported in 2015 found that 14.1% of substantiated child maltreatment victims reported having a disability (Child Welfare Information Gateway, 2018). Table 3.1 shows various estimates of the risk of maltreatment for children with disabilities. Additionally, the data are further complicated by the emerging understanding that there may be a

Table 3.1 Estimates of risk of child maltreatment

Finding	Source
11% of child maltreatment victims had a reported disability.	U.S. Department of Health and Human Services, Administration for Children and Families, Administration on Children, Youth and Families, Children's Bureau. (2010). Child Maltreatment 2009.
Children with a disability are 1.68 times more likely to experience abuse or neglect than children without a disability.	U.S. Department of Health and Human Services, Administration for Children and Families, Administration on Children, Youth and Families, Children's Bureau. (2006). Child Maltreatment 2004.
Children with an indication of disability are 1.5 times more likely to experience substantiated maltreatment 2 years after their first report.	Fluke, J. D., Shusterman, G. R., Hollinshead, D. M., & Yuan, Y. T. (2008). Longitudinal analysis of repeated child abuse reporting and victimization: Multistate analysis of associated factors. Child Maltreatment, 13(1), 76–88
Children with disabilities have overall lower rates of maltreatment compared to the general population but are 1.5 times more likely to be seriously harmed by the abuse or neglect they experience.	Sedlak, A. J., Mettenburg, J., Basena, M., Petta, I., McPherson, K., Greene, A., & Li, S. (2010). Fourth national incidence study of child abuse and neglect (NIS–4): Report to congress. Washington, DC: U.S. Department of Health and Human Services, Administration for Children and Families.
Children with a behavioral health condition who were maltreated before age 3 were 10 times more likely to be maltreated again.	Jaudes, P. K., & Mackey-Bilaver, L. (2008). Do chronic conditions increase young children's risk of being maltreated? Child abuse and neglect: The International Journal, 32(3), 671–681
Children with disabilities are 3.4 times more likely to be maltreated than children without disabilities.	Sullivan, P. M., & Knutson, J. F. (2000). Maltreatment and disabilities: A population-based epidemiological study. Child Abuse and Neglect, 24(10), 1257–1273

Adapted from "The Risk and Prevention of Maltreatment of Children with Disabilities" by Child Welfare Information Gateway, Bulletin for Professionals, March 2012

relationship between the increased risk and the type of disability, making an accurate estimate of the increased risk of maltreatment even more complex.

A groundbreaking 2011 study by Turner et al. provides a comprehensive framework from which to further understand the risk relationship among types of disability and forms of maltreatment (Turner, Vanderminden, Finkelhor, Hamby, & Shattuck, 2011). Spherically, Turner and colleagues' framework allows for a more refined understanding of the risk to children with disabilities of child sexual abuse. A full discussion of each type of disability and its relationship to various forms of maltreatment is beyond the scope of this chapter, but based on a nationally representative sample of 4046 children aged 2–17 years of age, Turner and colleagues' work has demonstrated in a compelling way that some children with disabilities are at greater risk for sexual victimization (Turner et al., 2011). Key to understanding this work is the notion of disabilities associated with externalizing behaviors versus those associated with internalizing behaviors. Externalizing behaviors are described as including disruptiveness, aggression, and being argumentative whereas internalizing behaviors are associated with classic symptoms of appearing depressed or withdrawn and being anxious and may manifest as crying easily, being socially withdrawn, and submitting to those who are aggressive. In the Turner et al. study, those children who had disabilities characterized by internalizing behaviors had a substantially higher risk for child maltreatment in general and had particularly higher risk for sexual victimization (Turner et al., 2011). Clinically, this finding would be consistent with earlier clinical studies which suggested that those children with disabilities that had behaviors that suggested emotional vulnerability (i.e., internalizing) that could be manipulated or coerced into silence about the abuse by the perpetrator might be at the highest risk. Other studies have shown that children with milder impairments, such as learning disabilities or communication and/or sensory impairments, are at greater risk for maltreatment than those with more severe impairments (Child Welfare Information Gateway, 2012). These various studies "underscore the importance of rejecting the use of a global idea of 'disability' in research; there are nuances in the type of abuse children experience in relation to their disability" (Child Welfare Information Gateway, 2012). In addition to the type of disability, other risk factors for child maltreatment include social, familial/parental, and institutional/caregiving factors which are briefly described in Table 3.2.

Responding to this growing awareness that some children with disabilities are at an increased risk for various forms of child maltreatment, there have been increasing calls to design, implement, and evaluate effective prevention and response programs directed at these special children. First steps include educating parents and families about the potential risks and ways to respond, adopting policies at the community and institutional level that make it difficult for a perpetrator to have unsupervised access to those who are vulnerable, and finally, when possible, educating children with disabilities about the risk and how they can help reduce that risk to themselves and to others around them. While the adults and community surrounding children with disabilities are responsible to protect these children and to prevent child maltreatment, there is likely value in alerting children to the reality of risk that may be in their environment and, in a developmentally appropriate manner, to help them avoid or reduce that risk. Table 3.3 outlines a number of promising practices related to child-focused prevention efforts.

3.3.2   Conclusion

The data are clearer and clearer that children with disabilities are at higher risk of child maltreatment. After decades of study, however, the nuances among type of disability and form of maltreatment are becoming clearer as well. Specifically related to risk of child sexual abuse, those children with disabilities that manifest with a constellation of internalizing behaviors seem to be at the highest risk. However, all children, those with and those without disabilities or special healthcare needs, ought to have comprehensive prevention efforts to protect them from all

Table 3.2 Additional risk factors beyond type of disability

Domain	Description and Citation
Social	• When children with disabilities are separated from their peers, it makes them seem "different" and unworthy of the same social or educational opportunities (Steinberg, M. A., & Hylton, J. R. (1998). *Responding to maltreatment of children with disabilities: A trainer's guide*. Portland, OR: Oregon Institute on Disability and Development, Child Development & Rehabilitation Center, Oregon Health Sciences University) • By devaluing the contributions of children with disabilities to society, it becomes more acceptable to treat them poorly or use violence (Sobsey, D. (1994). *Violence and abuse in the lives of people with disabilities: The end of silent acceptance?* Baltimore, MD: Paul H. Brookes Publishing Co.; Steinberg, M. A., & Hylton, J. R. (1998). *Responding to maltreatment of children with disabilities: A trainer's guide*. Portland, OR: Oregon Institute on Disability and Development, Child Development & Rehabilitation Center, Oregon Health Sciences University) • The belief that caregivers would never harm children with disabilities results in lack of attention to the problem (Sobsey, D. (1994). *Violence and abuse in the lives of people with disabilities: The end of silent acceptance?* Baltimore, MD: Paul H. Brookes Publishing Co.) • When children with disabilities are viewed as asexual, it may lead caregivers to deny them sex education that could help prevent abuse (Steinberg, M. A., & Hylton, J. R. (1998). *Responding to maltreatment of children with disabilities: A trainer's guide*. Portland, OR: Oregon Institute on Disability and Development, Child Development & Rehabilitation Center, Oregon Health Sciences University) • Children with disabilities who internalize societal attitudes toward disability may feel shame or feel less worthy of being treated respectfully (National Resource Center on Child Sexual Abuse, NCCAN. (1994). Responding to sexual abuse of children with disabilities: Prevention, investigation, and treatment. In *National Symposium on Abuse and Neglect of Children with Disabilities: Advance Literature*. National Center on Child Abuse and Neglect) • A lack of training impacts the ability of social workers, teachers, and other professionals to identify and report suspected maltreatment of children with disabilities (Hibbard, R. A., & Desch, L. W. (2007). Maltreatment of children with disabilities. *Pediatrics*, 119(5), 1018–1025; Kenny, M. (2004). Teachers' attitudes toward and knowledge of child maltreatment. *Child Abuse and Neglect*, 28(12), 1311–1319; Manders, J. E., & Stoneman, Z. (2009). Children with disabilities in the child protective services system: An analog study of investigation and case management. *Child Abuse and Neglect*, 33(4), 229–237)

(continued)

Table 3.2 (continued)

Domain	Description and Citation
Familial/ parental	• The family views the child as "different," sees the disability as an embarrassment, or mourns the loss of a "normal" child (Burrell, B., Thompson, B., & Sexton, D. (1994). Predicting child abuse potential across family types. *Child Abuse and Neglect*, 18(12), 1039–1049; Rycus, J. S., & Hughes, R. C. (1998). *Field guide to child welfare, Volume III: Child development and child welfare*. Washington, DC: Child Welfare League of America) • The parent lacks the skills, resources, or supports to respond to the child's special needs and provide adequate care or supervision (Ammerman, R. T., & Baladerian, N. J. (1993). *Maltreatment of children with disabilities*. National Committee to Prevent Child Abuse; Fisher, M. H., Hodapp, R. M., & Dykens, E. M. (2008). Child abuse among children with disabilities: What we know and what we need to know. *International review of research in mental retardation*, 35, 251–289; Hibbard, R. A., & Desch, L. W. (2007). Maltreatment of children with disabilities. *Pediatrics*, 119(5), 1018–1025) • The parent is unaware that his or her child with disabilities is at greater risk of maltreatment and may be unprepared to identify and protect the child from risky situations (Johnson, H. (2011). *Awareness and prevention of abuse/ neglect as experienced by children with disabilities*. Presented at the Council for Exceptional Children National Convention, National Harbor, MD) • The parent of a child who exhibits challenging behaviors may be more likely to exert unnecessary control or use physical punishment which may lead to the situation getting out of control with subsequent physical abuse-related injury (Helton, J. J., & Cross, T. P. (2011). The relationship of child functioning to parental physical assault: Linear and curvilinear models. *Child Maltreatment*, 16(2), 1–11; Mandell, D. S., Walrath, C. M., Manteuffel, B., Sgro, G., & Pinto-Martin, J. A. (2005). The prevalence and correlates of abuse among children with autism served in comprehensive community-based mental health settings. *Child Abuse and Neglect: The International Journal*, 29(12), 1359–1372; Sedlak, A. J., Mettenburg, J., Basena, M., Petta, I., McPherson, K., Greene, A., & Li, S. (2010). *Fourth national incidence study of child abuse and neglect (NIS–4): Report to congress*. Washington, DC: U.S. Department of Health and Human Services, Administration for Children and Families) • The parent of a child with disabilities who is unresponsive, unaffectionate, or exhibits behavior problems may have difficulty forming a strong attachment with the child; frequent hospitalizations may also weaken the parent–child attachment (Ammerman, R. T., & Patz, R. J. (1996). Determinants of child abuse potential: Contribution of parent and child factors. *Journal of Clinical Child Psychology*, 25(3), 300–307; Sobsey, D. (1994). *Violence and abuse in the lives of people with disabilities: The end of silent acceptance?* Baltimore, MD: Paul H. Brookes Publishing Co.; Tomison, A. M. (1996). Child maltreatment and disability. *Issues in Child Abuse Prevention*, 7, 1–11) • The cost of ongoing treatment or care for a child with disabilities may put a financial strain on the family or affect parental job stability (Fisher, M. H., Hodapp, R. M., & Dykens, E. M. (2008). Child abuse among children with disabilities: What we know and what we need to know. *International review of research in mental retardation*, 35, 251–289; Washington, L. (2009). A contextual analysis of caregivers of children with disabilities. *Journal of Human Behavior in the Social Environment*, 19(5), 554–571)

(continued)

Table 3.2 (continued)

Domain	Description and Citation
Institutional/ Caregiving	• An abusive subculture that allows for extreme power and control inequities between caregivers and children. • Dehumanization and detachment from the children. • Clustering vulnerable children with others who might harm them and tolerating inappropriate behavior among children. • Isolating children or allowing little to no outside contact. • Lack of procedures for reporting abuse or monitoring investigations of abuse (Sobsey, D. (1994). Violence and abuse in the lives of people with disabilities: The end of silent acceptance? Baltimore, MD: Paul H. Brookes Publishing Co.; Steinberg, M. A., & Hylton, J. R. (1998). Responding to maltreatment of children with disabilities: A trainer's guide. Portland, OR: Oregon Institute on Disability and Development, Child Development & Rehabilitation Center, Oregon Health Sciences University)

Adapted from "The Risk and Prevention of Maltreatment of Children with Disabilities" by Child Welfare Information Gateway, Bulletin for Professionals, March 2012

forms of maltreatment. Promising prevention practices that are emerging related to families, communities, institutions, and even the children themselves can best protect against the demonstrated risk of child maltreatment. Additional attention and effort are necessary to design, implement, and evaluate which practices are best suited to keep children with disabilities safe from the risk of maltreatment.

3.4 Risk of Child Sexual Abuse in Youth Serving Organizations

The term youth serving organizations (YSOs) is a descriptive term that refers to a wide range of nonfamilial entities where children and adolescents gather to pursue a variety of activities spanning faith-based organizations such as churches, synagogues, and mosques; sports-related teams and programs; and a broad array of more secular-oriented associations that seek to enhance skills, empower one's development, and explore a topic or issue in a deeper manner. While schools serve children and adolescents, they are often seen as separate and distinct from YSOs owing to public and private schools' centuries-long tradition of a professional connection to the education field and a clearly identifiable practice of local, state, and federal regulation and management replete with extensive policies and a host of standard operating procedures. At their best, YSOs provide opportunities for children and adolescents to grow, develop, and enjoy events and to engage in meaningful activities. At their worst however, YSOs may be a place for child maltreatment and sexual

Table 3.3 Child-focused prevention for children with disabilities and child maltreatment

Promising Practice	Description
Help children protect themselves.	Hold regular trainings to share information about abuse and neglect and talk about feelings children may experience if abuse is attempted. Help children understand how to identify it, respond to it, and tell others.
Teach children about their and others' bodies and sexuality.	Review the proper names for body parts and functions. Explain the difference between appropriate and inappropriate social or sexual behavior.
Reduce children's social isolation.	Ensure children with disabilities are included and feel welcome at all activities. Support them as they form and strengthen relationships with peers and trusted adults.
Maximize children's communication skills and tools.	Practice communication skills with them. Model healthy relationships and positive interactions with other children and adults.
Involve parents in their children's education.	Inform them when their children learn about abuse or sexuality; offer them the same training materials. Provide strategies for parents to reinforce the lessons at home.
Ensure prevention programs are inclusive and appropriate to children's ability levels, culture, and gender.	Remember that some children may need to be trained more frequently in order to retain the information.

Adapted from "The Risk and Prevention of Maltreatment of Children with Disabilities" by Child Welfare Information Gateway, Bulletin for Professionals, March 2012

abuse perpetrators to have ready access to vulnerable children whom they can victimize. Over the past several decades, the reality of this potential threat has become more apparent, fueled mainly by news coverage such as the 2002 reports of clergy sexual abuse in Boston (The Boston Globe, 2002), the 2011 reports of a sexual abuse scandal involving the Penn State football program (NPR, 2012), and most recently the 2016 coverage of sexual abuse scandal that focused on USA-Gymnastics and the sports medicine physician Larry Nassar (Daniels, 2017). These YSOs, which have the potential to promote high-quality experiences for the children and adolescents who participate, missed the mark in creating a safe environment for the young people in their charge. Typically, once the issue comes to light, an independent review is commissioned, reports written with extensive lists of recommendations, and changes are put into place. The recommendations typically talk about creating a culture of safety and efforts are prescribed to educate and raise awareness among both the adults and children involved in the institution, and efforts are made to generate policies and procedures that will help leaders and staff in those YSOs to organize and manage the environment in as safe a manner as possible. The overall goal is that children and adolescents are kept safe from child maltreatment and sexual victimization while participating in the YSOs' events and activities.

3.4.1 The Scope of the Problem

Data on the number of children who are maltreated while participating in YSOs is emerging. In 2016, Shattuck and colleagues reported on a combined analysis of three nationally representative surveys with a total of 13,052 children aged 0 to 17 years (Shattuck, Finkelhor, Turner, & Hamby, 2016). As expected, the vast majority of child maltreatment in this nationally representative sample was associated with adults in the family, namely a lifetime prevalence rate of 11.4% and an incidence rate of 5.9% in the past year (Shattuck et al., 2016). The total child maltreatment prevalence and incidence rates for non-family adults but excluding those non-family adults associated with the YSOs was 5.9% for a lifetime and 3.3% over the past year (Shattuck et al., 2016). Finally, the proportion of children and adolescents who experienced any type of maltreatment by adults associated with the YSOs was a prevalence rate of 0.8% over their lifetime and an incidence of 0.4% in the past year (Shattuck et al., 2016). While these rates are comparatively small, it did account for 105 YSO survivors of child maltreatment in this nationally representative sample of 13,052 children and provides a rigorously collected sample from which to learn more about the types of abuse to which children and adolescents are exposed while participating in YSO events and activities. Again, while comparatively small when considering YSOs, Shattuck and colleagues calculated that this 0.8% prevalence rate could represent approximately 36,000 cases of YSO-related child maltreatment (Shattuck et al., 2016).

Among YSO child maltreatment survivors, the most common form of maltreatment was verbal abuse, comprising 63.2% of survivors, followed by physical abuse, reported by 34.6% of survivors, sexual abuse at 6.4%, and then neglect at 0.8% (Shattuck et al., 2016).

3.4.2 Response and Prevention

Responding to the growing concern about YSO child maltreatment and prioritizing the design and adoption of effective organizational policies and procedures, in 2004 the Centers for Disease Control and Prevention (CDC) assembled an expert panel of child advocates, child sexual abuse researchers, prevention specialists, and YSO leaders who had child sexual abuse prevention programs. The CDC issued a comprehensive report in 2007 entitled, "Preventing Child Sexual Abuse Within Youth-serving Organizations: Getting Started on Policies and Procedures" (Saul & Audage, 2007) that sought to strike a balance between caution and caring related to the core work of YSOs along with the recognition that risk does exist. In the words of the report:

> The same dynamics that create a nurturing environment, and may ultimately protect against child sexual abuse, can also open the doors to sexually abusive behaviors. Research has shown that youth who are emotionally insecure, needy, and unsupported may be more

vulnerable to the attentions of offenders. By promoting close and caring relationships between youth and adults, organizations can help youth feel supported and loved and thus reduce their risk of child sexual abuse. But that same closeness between a youth and an adult can also provide the opportunity for abuse to occur. When developing policies for child sexual abuse prevention, organizations must balance the need to keep youth safe with the need to nurture and care for them. (Saul & Audage, 2007)

The CDC report articulates six components that ought to be addressed in a comprehensive set of policies and procedures directed at child sexual abuse prevention. Table 3.4 describes each component.

In addition to policies and procedures, educating and raising awareness of both the adults serving in the YSO organizations as well as the children served by the YSOs is viewed as an essential element of a comprehensive child maltreatment prevention program. The adult volunteers and staff need to learn about the problem of child maltreatment and how best to create and maintain an organizational culture that (1) recognizes the risk and (2) acts effectively to reduce and eliminate that risk. The children served need to know about the potential risk in a developmentally appropriate manner and how best to report concerns or the occurrence of actual

Table 3.4 Components of a comprehensive set of CSA Prevention policies and procedures

Component/goal	Critical strategies
Screening and selecting employees and volunteers *Goal: To select the best possible people for staff and volunteer positions and to screen out individuals who have sexually abused youth or are at risk to abuse.*	• Education about your organization and youth protection policies: By letting applicants know your organization is serious about protecting youth, you may deter some people at risk of abusing youth from applying for staff or volunteer positions. – Inform applicants about your organization's policies and procedures relevant to child sexual abuse prevention. – Share your code of conduct or ethics. – Require applicants to sign a document describing the policies and procedures of your organization to demonstrate their understanding and agreement. – Ask applicants if they have a problem with any of the policies and procedures. • Written application: The written application provides the information you need to assess the background and interests of applicants. Questions should help you determine whether applicants have mature, adult relationships as well as clear boundaries and ethical standards for their conduct with youth. • Personal interview: The personal interview provides an opportunity to meet applicants, determine if they are a good fit for your organization, and ask additional questions to screen for child sexual abuse risk factors. • Reference checks: These provide additional information about applicants and help verify previous work and volunteer history. • Criminal background checks: Background checks are an important tool in screening and selection. However, they have limitations. Criminal background checks will not identify most sexual offenders because most have not been caught. When this report was published, an efficient, effective, and affordable national background screening system was not available.

(continued)

Table 3.4 (continued)

Component/goal	Critical strategies

Guidelines on interactions between individuals
 Goal: To ensure the safety of youth in their interactions with employees/ volunteers and with each other.
	• Appropriate/inappropriate/harmful behaviors: Appropriate, positive interactions among youth and between employees/volunteers and youth are essential in supporting positive youth development, making youth feel valued, and providing the caring connections that serve as protective factors for youth. Conversely, inappropriate or harmful interactions put youth at risk for adverse physical and emotional outcomes. Organizations should identify behaviors that fall into the categories of appropriate, inappropriate, and harmful.
	 • Ratios of employees/volunteers to youth: The goal of setting ratios for the numbers of employees/volunteers to youth is to ensure the safety of the youth. There is no standard ratio for all situations. When making decisions about ratios, consider contextual variables such as:
	     – Age and developmental level of youth and employees/volunteers. If youth or employees/volunteers are young, you may need a lower ratio, that is, fewer youth per adult.
	     – Risk of the activity. Does it involve a great deal of isolation from others?
	     – Location of the activity. Is it in a classroom that is easy to monitor or at a park, where it is easier to lose track of individuals?
	 • One-on-one interactions: Some organizations have a policy to limit one-on-one interactions between youth and adults (i.e., having at least two adults present at all times with youth). The goal of such a policy is to prevent the isolation of one adult and one youth, a situation that elevates the risk for child sexual abuse. This strategy must be modified based on the mission of your organization. Limit one-on-one interactions whenever possible by having at least two adults present at all times with youth. Choose one of three options relating to this policy:
	     – Make this a mandatory policy at all times.
	     – Make this policy dependent on the risk of the activity or situation, such as overnight trips.
	     – Maintain other safeguards such as extra supervision or contact with youth and employees/volunteers and more stringent screening if the mission of your organization requires one-on-one time between employees/volunteers and youth (e.g., mentoring programs).
	 • Risk of interactions between youth: Your organization needs to address interactions among youth in addition to monitoring interactions between employees/volunteers and youth. Many strategies that focus on the interactions between employees/volunteers and youth can be tailored to address interactions among youth.
	 • Prohibitions and restrictions on certain activities: Some activities, such as hazing and secret ceremonies, overnight trips, bathing, changing, bathroom interactions, and nighttime activities, pose greater risks for child sexual abuse. Prohibiting or restricting such activities will depend largely on the context of your organization.
	 • Out-of-program contact restrictions: There are two types of out-of-program contact restrictions. The first type involves the contact of youth with employees/volunteers outside the context of the program. Your organization should limit contact between employees/volunteers and youth to organization-sanctioned activities and programs and/ or to certain locations, such as activities within your organization's building. The second type is contact between youth and people not affiliated with your organization that occurs while youth are under the care of your organization.
	 • Caregiver information and permission: Your organization should obtain addresses and contact information for youth and caregivers (i.e., parents and guardians). This information should never be released to unauthorized individuals. Your organization also should obtain permission from caregivers for youth to participate in certain activities, such as field trips, late-night activities, and overnight trips.
	 • Responsibility for youth: Your organization should clarify when it is responsible for youth and when caregivers are responsible.

(continued)

Table 3.4 (continued)

Component/goal	Critical strategies

Monitoring behavior *Goal: To prevent, recognize, and respond to inappropriate and harmful behaviors and to reinforce appropriate behaviors.*	• Responding to what is observed: Your organization must be prepared to respond to interactions among youth and between employees/volunteers and youth.
	 • Develop a monitoring protocol so that employees/volunteers are clear about their roles and responsibilities. Employees/volunteers should be prepared to respond immediately to inappropriate or harmful behavior, potential risk situations, and potential boundary violations.
	   – Enforce the protocol so that appropriate actions follow. Supervisors need to redirect inappropriate behaviors to promote positive behaviors, confront inappropriate or harmful behaviors, and report these behaviors if necessary.
	 • Roles and responsibilities: All employees/volunteers should be responsible for monitoring behavior and interactions within your organization. Everyone needs to know how and what to monitor. Define roles and responsibilities by including monitoring within a job description, specifying what employees/volunteers need to do from the very beginning, and providing training.
	 • Clear reporting structure within organization: Your organization should have a well-defined reporting structure so people know who to contact if they observe potentially inappropriate or harmful behavior.
	   – Require employees/volunteers to report any behaviors and practices that may be harmful.
	   – Establish direct-line and back-up reporting systems within your organization. The back-up option should be used if the incident involves the direct-line authority.
	   – Create a climate that encourages people to question confusing or uncertain behaviors and practices.
	 • Observation and contact with employees/volunteers: Your organization should use multiple monitoring methods to get a clear picture of how individuals are interacting.
	   – Use formal supervision, including regular evaluations.
	   – Use informal supervision, including regular and random observation (e.g., roving and checking interactions throughout an activity period), and maintain frequent contact with employees/volunteers and youth who interact off-site.
	 • Documentation that monitoring has occurred: Although it may be clear when other child sexual abuse prevention strategies, such as screening or environmental policies, have been implemented in your organization, it is harder to be sure that adequate monitoring is occurring. Documenting that monitoring has occurred emphasizes to employees/volunteers that it is an essential, nonnegotiable part of your organization's child sexual abuse prevention efforts.

Ensuring safe environments *Goal: To keep youth from situations in which they are at increased risk for sexual abuse.*	• Visibility: Building or choosing spaces that are open and visible to multiple people can create an environment where individuals at risk for sexually abusive behaviors do not feel comfortable abusing. • Privacy when toileting, showering, changing clothes: Your organization should develop policies and procedures for reducing risk during activities such as toileting, showering, and changing clothes that consider not just the risk of employee/volunteer sexual abuse, but also the risk of inappropriate or harmful contact among youth. • Access control: Your organization should monitor who is present at all times. • Off-site activity guidelines: Your organization should define and communicate its on-site and off-site physical boundaries. • Transportation policies: Your organization should define who is responsible for transporting youth to and from regular activities and special events (e.g., field trips, overnight trips).

(continued)

Table 3.4 (continued)

Component/goal	Critical strategies

Responding to inappropriate behavior, breaches in policy, and allegations and suspicions of child sexual abuse *Goal: To respond quickly and appropriately to (1) inappropriate or harmful behavior, (2) infractions of child sexual abuse prevention policies, and (3) evidence or allegations of child sexual abuse.*	What to respond to within the organization and what to report to the authorities: It is often difficult to find the balance between being vigilant and protective of youth and being so hypervigilant that the positive parts of programs (e.g., relationships between adults and youth) are lost. In responding, the need for this balance involves recognizing the tension between over-reacting and under-reacting.
	• Reporting process: If evidence of child sexual abuse has surfaced or an allegation has been made, a formal report needs to be made to an outside agency. Ensure that your organization's reporting policies are consistent with current state law.
	  – Who must report.
	  – To whom to report.
	  – When to report.
	• Internal records: Although your organization should not investigate allegations or suspicions of child sexual abuse in lieu of reporting them to the authorities, it should develop a system to track allegations and suspicions of child sexual abuse cases.
	• Confidentiality policy: Because of the sensitive nature of child sexual abuse cases, your organization should decide in advance what information should remain private and what information can be made public.
	• Response to the press and the community: Your organization should decide on a strategy for responding to the press and the community before an allegation has been made.
	  – Designate a spokesperson for questions and inquiries.
	  – Have employees/volunteers go through training on how to deal with the press and the community.
	• Membership/employment of alleged offenders: Remember that an allegation of child sexual abuse does not equate to guilt. The person alleged to have engaged in sexually abusive behavior should not be labeled as an offender or sexual abuser. However, once a suspicion or allegation has been communicated, it needs to be reported to the authorities, and your organization must take certain steps to protect the youth under its care. A decision must be made whether to suspend membership or employment.

Training about child sexual abuse prevention *Goal: To give people information and skills to help them prevent and respond to child sexual abuse.*	Integration of content into the entire organization: • Ensure that training content is modeled by everyone in your organization, from management to employees/volunteers. • Training content should be evident in performance measures, supervisors' feedback to employees/volunteers, caregivers' observations, and treatment of youth by your organization. • Meld elements of your organization's philosophy or mission with the child sexual abuse training. For example, a faith-based organization may want to incorporate elements of its faith into the training content.

Adapted from *Preventing Child Sexual Abuse Within Youth-Serving Organizations: Getting Started on Policies and Procedures* by J. Saul and N.C. Audage, 2007, Centers for Disease Control and Prevention, National Center for Injury Prevention and Control, Atlanta, GA

abuse. In 2012, the Safe Environment Work Group of the United States Conference of Catholic Bishops commissioned the child policy organization Children at Risk to draft a white paper (some of which were published in a subsequent topical review) that would summarize the literature around the child educational and training elements of safe environment training oriented towards the prevention of child sexual abuse (Desai & Lew, 2012; Giardino, Desai, Lew, Doerr, & Nojadera, 2016). In short, the white paper observed that over 20 years of research on child-focused sexual abuse prevention programs showed that prevention programs were effective at increasing children's knowledge about sexual abuse, increasing the reporting of past and current abuse, and teaching children self-protection skills (Desai & Lew,

2012; Giardino et al., 2016). Specifically, Topping and Barron (2009) were cited as determining that after safe environment training efforts, children felt more self-confident and assertive, felt less anxious because they knew how to respond to unsafe situations and felt encouraged to dialogue with parents about unsafe situations. Finkelhor (2009) observed that safe environment training discouraged self-blame in the event of abuse and that in the event of abuse, children were more likely to feel that they were able to protect themselves and to prevent the situation from getting worse. Owing to methodological issues, the various child-focused safe environment programs could not be definitively shown to decrease the incidence of child sexual abuse, however. A number of curricular best practices were identified from the literature summarized in the commissioned white paper, and they are shown in Table 3.5.

3.4.3   Conclusion

As seen from both the CDC report and Desai white paper described above, a number of best practices or promising practices exist to help make the environments of children safe from the risk of child maltreatment in general and child sexual abuse in specific. A combination of efforts directed at (1) education and awareness building and (2) sound policies and procedures will be necessary to design, implement, and monitor in YSO organizations so that the risk of YSO child maltreatment is reduced and eliminated. The Children's Bureau's Child Welfare Information Gateway suggests six promising practices related to the prevention of nonfamilial maltreatment that are applicable to the discussion of YSO-related child maltreatment:

Promising Practices for the Prevention of Child Maltreatment in Nonfamilial Settings

- Carefully screen job applicants for experience working with children with disabilities and for prior reports of maltreatment.
- Train staff in positive behavior management techniques that limit the use of restraint or seclusion.
- Maintain effective staff/child ratios and set realistic expectations for staff responsibilities.
- Provide strong supervision and support that emphasize a culture of child protection and relationship-building between staff and children.
- Establish procedures and staff training on how to identify and report suspected maltreatment.
- Ensure an open environment that welcomes families and allows for unannounced checks by external reviewers.

Reprinted from "The Risk and Prevention of Maltreatment of Children with Disabilities" by Child Welfare Information Gateway, Bulletin for Professionals, March 2012.

The CDC report on YSOs and child sexual abuse prevention ends on an aspirational note in a section entitled "Moving Forward" recognizing the challenge inherent in such a massive task along with the recognition that prevention of child maltreatment is possible. In the words of the report:

> Implementing a child sexual abuse prevention policy and making the changes necessary to protect youth from child sexual abuse in organizations are not easy tasks. Although organizations should take on as many individual strategies to prevent child sexual abuse as they are able, organizations must have a strong infrastructure in place to serve as a foundation for efforts to prevent child sexual abuse … If your organization is committed to preventing child sexual abuse and takes this charge on thoughtfully and with careful planning, it can and will succeed in creating a safer place for the youth under its care. (Saul & Audage, 2007)

3.5   Online Sexual Solicitations of Minors

Reena Isaac

3.5.1   Introduction

The development of the Internet and other digital technologies in the last few decades have changed how people, especially adolescents, communicate, entertain, and interact with new media. The Internet has now become a fully integrated component of the lives of adolescents.

When Pew Research Center began tracking social media adoption in 2005, just 5% of American adults used at least one of these platforms. By 2011 that share had risen to half of all Americans, and today more than 69% of the public uses some type of social media (Pew Research Center, 2017). In 2016, 78% of Americans had a social media profile, representing a 5% growth compared to the previous year (Statista Research Department, 2019). Fifty-eight percent of American teens have downloaded an app to a cell phone or tablet (Madden, Lenhart, Cortesi, & Gasser, 2013). With the rapid pace of penetration of Internet-enabled devices (e.g., computers, laptops, smartphones, and tablets) and online communication services, such as social media networks and social applications, it would likely follow that digital technologies might serve as a tool for those seeking to connect with and solicit minors for sexual purposes.

Table 3.5 Best practices in CSA safe environment training

Best practices in implementation		Best practices in curriculum	
Frequency	• Begin at a young age. • At least four sessions per year. • Repeated for several years.	Knowledge	• Definition of child sexual abuse. • How to recognize abuse. • How common abuse is. • Dangers of the internet. • How to identify potential abusers. • Abusers can be family members, friends, or acquaintances.
Pedagogical methods	• Modeling. • Group discussion. • Role-playing.	Body ownership	• Difference between appropriate and inappropriate touches.
Instructors	• Designed to be taught by a range of presenters. • Instructor training, with particular attention on how to respond to reports of abuse.	Self-protection skills	• How to say no. • Strategies to avoid abuse.
Parents	• Active parental involvement in training.	Mental health	• Discourage self-blame in case of abuse.
Evaluation	• Evaluations built into program.	Disclosure	• Importance of reporting past or current abuse. • Recognition of common barriers to disclosure. • Train victims to tell trusted adult. • Train friends of victims to disclose and promote disclosure.

3.5.2 Unique Qualities of Internet Cases

The scope of Internet-related crimes against children has been characterized by two features: rapid growth and changing dynamics (Mitchell, Jones, Finkelhor, & Wolak, 2011). Arrests of online sex crime perpetrators (i.e., sex offenders who used the Internet or related technologies to meet victims) increased more than threefold between 2000 and 2006 (Wolak, Finkelhor, & Mitchell, 2009).

Along with the rapid growth in cases leading to arrests during that time period, new and evolving tactics by offenders circulated. The use of video, for example, increased over the years as webcams were rarely used in the course of these crimes in 2000. By 2006, however, among offenders arrested for an online sex crime against an actual youth, 27% used video communications to interact with victims (Wolak et al., 2009). Offenders who seek to commercially profit and exploit minors are adept at quickly adopting the newer Internet technologies given their certain advantages. The vast reach and sheer speed of the Internet allow for it to be an efficient means of reaching large and varied groups such as targeted pools of victims for traffickers, deviants with extreme tastes, or those seeking access to children, and those searching for child pornography. Online offenders may seek the corners of the Internet as a clandestine means to hide their activities, such as in encrypting communications and picture files and using wireless technologies that may be difficult to trace to specific locations and users (Mitchell et al., 2011).

The immense popularity of social networking sites (SNSs) among both adults and the younger population and the many media news reports of online predators using SNSs have raised concerns for the safety of today's youth. Offenders of online sex crimes have used SNSs along various lines for varied purposes (Mitchell, Finkelhor, Jones, & Wolak, 2010). One national study of arrests for Internet-related sex crimes against minors noted SNSs to have been used to initiate relationships in 50% of victim-involved cases (Mitchell et al., 2010). In this same study, such cases involved the communication between the offender and victim through messages on both the victims' (98%) and offenders' (94%) SNSs. SNSs were also used to disseminate information or pictures of the victim. Such cases often involved offenders who were accessing information about the victim such as determining the victim's interests (82%), home or school (65%), whereabouts at a specific time (26%), and viewing photos of the victim (81%). SNSs are largely used in undercover operations in which investigators set up web pages and profiles in the pretense of being minors online. In the Mitchell study, most of these cited cases were initiated in chat rooms (82%), 7% were initiated through the investigator's SNSs, 1% through the offender's. The remaining cases were initiated through other online access (e.g., instant messaging, online want ads) (Mitchell et al., 2010).

3.5.3 Offender Characteristics/Demographics

Negative and unwanted sexual experiences facilitated through digital technologies can be divided into three categories of behaviors. Sexual coercion or "sextortion" may manifest through blackmail, bribery, or threats such as demanding that the victim perform either online or in-person sex acts or provide the release of sexual images. Another type of such negative online experience is the use of digital technologies to manifest a live sexual contact, such as the use of a dating or "hook up" app to organize a physical meeting with a victim before then sexually assaulting them. The third category includes the use of technologies to solicit and arrange a third party to sexually assault a person (Henry & Powell, 2016).

While the individual and collective circumstances of negative sexual online experiences are daunting and well portrayed in the media, analysis of such cases as they relate to minors through available current studies provide a broader lens and clearer perspective to the issue. From data from a national sample of law enforcement agencies about Internet-related sex crimes against minors, and detailed telephone interviews with investigators about individual cases, it was observed that compared with know-in-person offenders, online-meeting offenders were less likely to have criminal backgrounds, including problems with drugs or alcohol, histories of violent behavior, and prior arrests for nonsexual offenses (Wolak & Finkelhor, 2013). The majority of cases in both groups involved statutory rape (i.e., nonforcible illegal sexual activity with underage youth) or noncontact offenses such as child pornography production or sexual solicitation of a minor (Wolak & Finkelhor, 2013). Force or coercion were rare; most victims were adolescents and girls; and most arrested offenders were young men.

More offenders and victims who met in SNSs did not exclusively use SNSs as their form of communication as they also communicated by text messaging through cell phone and email compared with those who met in other online venues. Cases that involved SNSs in some capacity were more likely to result in a face-to-face meeting than cases not involving SNSs. However, this finding could be a result of the older age of victims and younger age of offenders in SNS cases. It is likely that aspects of SNSs themselves may contribute to this, by providing much exchange of information to both the victim and offender, the victim may feel more comfortable and less inhibited in arranging such a meeting, given the perception of familiarity with the offender based on the information received (Wolak & Finkelhor, 2013).

Most online-meeting offenders target adolescents and perpetrate nonforcible crimes involving illegal sexual contact with youth who are too young to consent to sexual activity (statutory rape) (Wolak & Finkelhor, 2013). Promises of love and romance to seduce victims or target adolescents who are looking for sexual experiences are not exclusive to online offenders. Of note, most perpetrators of nonforcible sex crimes against children and adolescents do not meet victims online; they know them in-person prior to the offense.

3.5.4 The Declining Trend in Online Sexual Solicitation of Minors

In 2010, 1 in 10 youth reported receiving an unwanted sexual solicitation, a 50% reduction in rates when compared with one in 5 youth who reported such an experience when the YISS was conducted in 2000 (Jones, Mitchell, & Finkelhor, 2012). The trends in unwanted experiences online may oppose conventional thoughts that the general population, health professionals, and the media have about the realities of online solicitations of minors.

The reason for the steady decline in rates may be due to several factors. It is possible that online behavior by minors has changed in ways that reduce such solicitations. Changes in online communication preferences were noted in that (1) youth have migrated from chat rooms to social networking environments, (2) youth may be restricting more of their interactions to people they know, thereby resulting in a reduction in online unwanted sexual comments or requests. It is also possible that young people have become more cautious regarding who they interact with because of Internet safety education. A tremendous effort has been made over the last several years to warn young people about the dangers of online sexual interactions.

While an overall downward trend of youth Internet users who received online limited sexual solicitations was observed between 2000 and 2005, a slightly larger percentage of youth Internet users experienced aggressive sexual solicitations during the same time period (Mitchell, Finkelhor, & Wolak, 2007). These solicitations include an increased risk for offline criminal victimization. While enhanced online education and prevention trainings may have deterred the casual solicitor, the more resolute and determined solicitors will persist in their attempts to interface online with victims. Additionally, it may be that prevention messages have not penetrated a higher risk segment of young Internet users.

3.5.5 Prevention

Adolescents are a fickle group as they select, switch, and blend various platforms for entertainment and communication in the ever-changing seas of social media and networking sites. This pace of change poses a tremendous challenge to parents and healthcare providers. By the time the dynamics of one particular online environment are fully understood, that environment may have changed so completely that intervention and prevention strategies are obsolete. It is this combination of mercurial use of social media by youth with the quickly changing online landscape that supports the targeting of adolescent behaviors instead of specific online locations where the Internet-related crimes occur (Ybarra & Mitchell, 2008). Research suggests that most victims of such Internet sex crimes often know that they are meeting the offender for sex and may re-engage in the practice (Wolak, Finkelhor, & Kimberly, 2008). Therefore, shifting the focus of prevention messages to helping adolescents make mature, thoughtful, and safer choices about sex and relationships rather than alarming them of the less likely scenario of the lurid adult stalker and potential abduction situation as depicted so often by the media would provide a greater reach and impact. By highlighting recommended behaviors, such as refraining from talking about sex with people they meet online and not posting sexual images of themselves, they can take this knowledge with them online, regardless of whatever new technology becomes the next popular item in the dynamic online landscape.

3.5.6   Future Research

Future research needs to focus on identifying the extent and nature of a range of online sexual crimes and behaviors, including prevalence and impacts of victimization and perpetration, and the gender dynamics of these behaviors as they relate to minors (Henry & Powell, 2016). Another area for exploration is the study of why the young participate in certain risky online behaviors such as talking about sex with and sending personal information including intimate photos to someone they met online. One recent study showed that sex-related online behaviors predicted poorer body and sexual self-perceptions among adolescents (Doornwaard et al., 2014). Future studies should examine whether adolescents with negative body and sexual self-perceptions selectively engage in sex-related online behaviors and thus are at increased risk for developing more negative self-perceptions.

3.6   Backlash Against Child Sexual Abuse

3.6.1   Introduction

Child sexual abuse is recognized as a serious, medical, public health, and social problem (Conte, 1994). As a topic of professional study, CSA has a relatively short history, being ushered into modern pediatric practice via a prominent invited lecture in 1977 by the legendary C Henry Kempe and published as an article in a prestigious journal, entitled "Sexual Abuse: Another Hidden Pediatric Problem." In that article, Kempe comments:

> Pediatrics started, about a hundred years ago, around the single critical issue of deaths due to diarrhea, caused by unsafe milk. Pediatrics has progressed to a comprehensive approach to child health… The modern pediatrician…will attempt to return the child to his normal and optimal state of health as soon as possible and to try to minimize the deleterious effects of illness on the normal growth and development of the child, from both the emotional and the physical point of view. I have chosen to speak on the subject of sexual abuse of children and adolescents as another hidden pediatric problem and a neglected area. More and more clinical problems related to sexual abuse come to our attention every year. In our training and in our practice, we pediatricians are insufficiently aware of the frequency of sexual abuse. (Kempe, 1978, p. 382)

Despite this relatively short history, a backlash against it emerged, and concerns about CSA and how it is identified, evaluated, and investigated have come under close professional and media scrutiny. The definition of a backlash varies. The Merriam-Webster dictionary defines backlash as a strong adverse reaction (Merriam-Webster, n.d.). In a public or political sense, a backlash arises when emerging changes to the status quo are perceived as threatening to a group that has power to resist that change, essentially when a sense emerges that a movement has gone too far and must be slowed or stopped to prevent further erosion or loss (Mansbridge & Shames 2008). As applied to the backlash against sexual abuse seen in the 1980s, news coverage documented a growing sense that child advocates where going too far, going about their work in the wrong way and being overzealous and too aggressive, and in short, falsely accusing innocent parents and other caregivers such as day care providers in their zeal to stamp out child sexual abuse around every corner. David Hechler in a 1988 text entitled "The Battle and the Backlash: The Child Sexual Abuse War" sums it up this way:

> One thing is clear; there is a war. There are those who feel that the country is suffering from an epidemic of child sexual abuse and those who feel that there is an epidemic all right, but not of sex abuse—of "sex accuse," as some have disparagingly called it. The pendulum has swung too far, they say, and what we see now is a blizzard of false accusations. (Hechler, 1988)

In 1992, a 2-day invitational conference entitled Defining and Responding to the Backlash Against Child Protection was held at the McGeorge School of Law at the University of the Pacific in Sacramento, California to explore a range of topics related to the backlash against CSA. The proceedings of this scholarly conference were published in a book by John E. B. Myers, JD, entitled "The Backlash: Child Protection Under Fire." Several of the insights developed and published from this conference are summarized in this chapter. In addition to scholarly publications from child advocates, media coverage is an important element to our understanding of how topics and issues are understood by both professional and lay audiences (Weatherred, 2015). Weatherred developed a timeline that calls out specific stages of news coverage of CSA: early history (1960–1979), backlash (1980–1989), sex-offender legislation in the US (1990–1999), religious institutions (2000–2009), and high-profile institutions (2010–present). The backlash stage was characterized by prominent day care center cases and the emergence of the so-called recovered memories of sexual victimization with the overriding message being a concern over false allegations harming the accused (Weatherred, 2015). The details of these scenarios are beyond the scope of this chapter, but the consensus that emerged at the backlash conference was that the adverse reaction was not directed towards protecting children from child sexual abuse; instead the reaction was directed at the entire child protection process which was perceived by some as functioning poorly and not achieving its aims. The end result was that the identification, evaluation, and investigation of suspected CSA cases by child protection professionals came under significant scrutiny.

3.6.2   The Backlash Context

Myers suggested that the field take the backlash seriously and draws the distinction between legitimate and illegitimate criticism. The child protection field does indeed experience its share of challenges, which includes staffing levels, timeliness of response, and occasional failures to protect children in foster care. Concerns about these challenges and others are legitimate, and the field should continually learn and improve. On the other hand, overly broad criticisms such as the "...blanket claim that thousands of families are accused of child abuse and as a result are permanently damaged..." seem overly reactive and would be considered illegitimate since "...no data exist documenting such horrible consequences in large numbers of cases" in this framework (Conte, 1994). What prompts the backlash against child sexual abuse? According to Myers (1994) the fuel behind the CSA backlash movement includes (1) strong emotions around sexual victimization, (2) blind spots about sexual abuse, and (3) faults in the child protection system. Finkelhor adds there is a cyclical nature of social movements, so the success of the child protection movement in capturing public attention around CSA in part allows for a reaction against it, especially when shortcomings in the practice of child protection emerge (Finkelhor, 1994). Child advocates involved in the child protection movement did in fact overstate their case, including (1) exaggerating statements of fact such as "children never lie about abuse," (2) failing to learn from legitimate criticism, and (3) demonstrating a tendency to let the zeal of protecting children get ahead of knowledge as seen in the daycare cases where poor interviewing techniques were employed (Meyers, 1994). Clearly, professional practice in child protection must evolve as research emerges to inform and refine best practices. Conte (1994) contends that child protection has a tradition of continually improving from a critical analysis of cases and being open to lessons learned. Specifically, Conte highlights one such example of improvement based on emerging research:

> ...We know and do things today that we could not envision a few years ago. We also believed things in the past that we know now were not accurate. To the extent that decisions were based on those ideas, it is likely that errors were made. For example, not all that long ago professionals believed that 'behavior proves abuse.' It was thought that certain childhood behaviors (such as fearfulness, nightmares, and acting younger than one's developmental age) were proof that the child had been abused. It is now generally acknowledged that these behaviors are indicative of stress or anxiety and not diagnostic of child abuse. Decisions based on the belief that a child had been sexually abused and interventions that arose from this belief may have been in error when based on the notion that "behavior proves abuse." (Conte, 1994)

3.6.3   Looking Towards the Future

Despite the at times extreme positions taken by those in the CSA movement and the frequent paucity of data to support the extreme positions, the child protection and Child Abuse Pediatrics fields need to be open to the valid criticism of clinical practice. The backlash revealed opportunities for improvement in the clinical arena, including the need for:

- Standardization of procedures around interviewing children suspected of having been abused.
- Professionalism to temper zeal among child advocates.

- Specialization among the professionals who conduct interviews, evaluations, and investigations of suspected CSA.
- Independence of "Evaluation" vs. "Investigation" with child health professionals conducting the evaluation and child protection and law enforcement professionals conducting the investigation.
- Reliance on emergence of evidence to guide continual improvement of best practice.

Finally, Conte offers words of wisdom for all professionals working with children and families confronting child sexual abuse:

> …professionals in the field of child sexual abuse must make every effort to assure that what they believe, what they know, and what they do is based on sound research evidence and works directly to improve the lives of abused children. Science is a demanding taskmaster which requires that knowledge be tested and demonstrated. Sexually abused children, and those who …influence their lives, deserve professional interventions that are based on well-established principles and ideas. (Conte, 1994 pp.230-231)

In sum, the best response to a backlash movement is to firmly ground clinical practice in rigorous, evidence-informed continuous improvement efforts.

References

Ahern, E. C., Stolzenberg, S. N., & Lyon, T. D. (2015). Do prosecutors use interview instructions or build rapport with child witnesses? *Behavioral Sciences & the Law, 33*(4), 476–492.

Alaggia, R. (2010). An ecological analysis of child sexual abuse disclosure: Considerations for child and adolescent mental health. *Journal of the Canadian Academy of Child and Adolescent Psychiatry, 19*, 32–39.

Alaggia, R., & Kirshenbaum, S. (2005). Speaking the unspeakable: Exploring the impact of family dynamics on child sexual abuse disclosures. *Families in Society, 86*, 227–234.

Allnock, D., & Miller, P. (2013). *No one noticed, no one heard: A study of disclosures in child abuse.* London, England: NSPCC.

Anderson, G. D. (2016). The continuum of disclosure: Exploring factors predicting tentative disclosure of child sexual abuse allegations during forensic interview and implications for practice, policy and future research. *J Child Sex Ab, 25*(4), 382–402.

Berlinger, L., & Conte, J. R. (1990). The process of victimization: The victims' perspective. *Child Abuse & Neglect, 14*, 29–40.

Berlinger, L., & Conte, J. R. (1995). The efforts of disclosure and intervention on sexually abused children. *Child Abuse & Neglect, 19*, 371–384.

Bethell, D. C., Blumberg, S. J., Stein, R. E., Strickland, B., Robertson, J., & Newacheck, P. W. (2015). Taking stock of the CSHCN screener: A review of common questions and current reflections. *Academic Pediatrics, 15*(2), 165–176. https://doi.org/10.1016/j.acap.2014.10.003.

Bicanic, I. A., Hehenkamp, L. M., van de Putte, E. M., van Wijk, A. J., & de Jongh, A. (2015). Predictors of delayed disclosure of rape in female adolescents and young adults. *European Journal of Psychotraumatology, 6.* https://doi.org/10.3402/ejpt.v6.25883.

Block, S. D., Foster, E. M., Pierce, M. W., Berkoff, M. C., & Runyan, D. K. (2013). Multiple forensic interviews during investigations of child sexual abuse: A cost-effectiveness analysis. *Applied Developmental Science, 17*(4), 174–183.

Bullock, M., Gelman, R., & Baillargeon, R. (1982). The development of causal reasoning. In W. J. Friedman (Ed.), *The developmental psychology of time* (pp. 209–254). New York, NY: Academic Press.

Bunting, L. (2008). Sexual offences against children: An exploration of attrition in the Northern Ireland criminal justice system. *Child Abuse & Neglect, 32*, 1109–1118.

Bussey, K. (1992). Lying and truthfulness: Children's definitions, standards, and evaluative reactions. *Child Development, 63*, 129–137.

Castelli, P., & Goodman, G. S. (2014). Children's perceived emotional behavior at disclosure and prosecutors' evaluations. *Child Abuse & Neglect, 38*, 1521–1532.

Ceci, S. J., & Friedman, R. D. (2000, November). The suggestibility of children: Scientific research and legal implications. *Cornell Law Review, 86*(1), 33–108.

Centers for Disease Control and Prevention, National Center on Birth Defects and Developmental Disabilities (CDC NCBDDD). (2019a). *Important milestones: Your child by three years.* Retrieved from https://www.cdc.gov/ncbddd/actearly/milestones/milestones-3yr.html

Centers for Disease Control and Prevention, National Center on Birth Defects and Developmental Disabilities (CDC NCBDDD). (2019b). *Important milestones: Your child by four years.* Retrieved from https://www.cdc.gov/ncbddd/actearly/milestones/milestones-4yr.html

Centers for Disease Control and Prevention, National Center on Birth Defects and Developmental Disabilities (CDC NCBDDD). (2019c). *Important milestones: Your child by five years.* Retrieved from https://www.cdc.gov/ncbddd/actearly/milestones/milestones-5yr.html

Centers for Disease Control and Prevention, National Center on Birth Defects and Developmental Disabilities (CDC NCBDDD). (2019d). *Middle childhood (9–11 years of age).* Retrieved from https://www.cdc.gov/ncbddd/childdevelopment/positiveparenting/middle2.html

Centers for Disease Control and Prevention, National Center on Birth Defects and Developmental Disabilities (CDC NCBDDD). (2019e). *Middle childhood (6–8 years of age).* Retrieved from https://www.cdc.gov/ncbddd/childdevelopment/positiveparenting/middle.html

Child Welfare Information Gateway. (2012). *The risk and prevention of maltreatment of children with disabilities.* Washington, DC: U.S. Department of Health and Human Services, Children's Bureau.

Child Welfare Information Gateway. (2018). *The risk and prevention of maltreatment of children with disabilities.* Washington, DC.: U.S. Department of Health and Human Services, Children's Bureau.

Collin-Vezina, D., De La Sablonniere-Griffin, M., Palmer, A. M., & Milne, L. (2015). A preliminary mapping of individual, relational, and social factors that impede disclosure of childhood sexual abuse. *Child Abuse & Neglect, 43*, 123–134.

Conte, J. R. (1994). Child sexual abuse: Awareness and backlash. *The Future of Children, 4*(2), 224–232.

Craven, S., Brown, S., & Gilchrist, E. (2006). Sexual grooming of children: Review of literature and theoretical considerations. *Journal of Sexual Aggression, 12*, 287–299.

Crisma, M., Bascelli, E., Paci, D., & Romito, P. (2004). Adolescents who experienced sexual abuse: Fears, needs, and impediments to disclosure. *Child Abuse & Neglect, 28*, 1035–1048.

Cyr, M., Frapper, J. Y., Hebert, M., Tourigny, M., McDuff, P., & Turcotte, M. E. (2016). Psychological and physical health of non-offending parents after disclosure of sexual abuse by their child. *J Child Sex Ab., 25*(7), 757–776.

Daniels, D. J., with assistance from Praesidium. (2017). *Report to USA gymnastics on proposed policy and procedural changes for the protection of young athletes.* Retrieved from https://usagym.org/PDFs/About%20USA%20Gymnastics/ddreport_062617.pdf

Davies, M., & Rogers, P. (2009). Perceptions of blame and credibility toward victims of childhood sexual abuse: Differences across victim age, victim-perpetrator relationship, and respondent gender in a depicted case. *Journal of Child Sexual Abuse, 18*, 78–92.

Desai, K., & Lew, D. (2012). *Safe environment training: The effectiveness of the Catholic Church's child sexual abuse prevention programs.* Children at Risk Institute. Retrieved from http://www.usccb.org/issues-and-action/child-and-youth-protection/upload/Safe-Environment-White-Paper-FINAL.pdf

Doornwaard, S., Bickham, D., Rich, M., Vanwesenbeeck, I., van den Eijnden, R., & ter Bogt, T. (2014). Sex-related online behaviors and adolescents' body and sexual self-perceptions. *Pediatrics, 134*, 1103–1110.

Finkelhor, D. (1990). Early and long-term effects of child sexual abuse: An update. *Professional Psychology: Research and Practice, 21*, 325–330.

Finkelhor, D. (1994). The backlash and the future of child protection advocacy: Insights from the study of social issues. In J. Myers (Ed.), *The backlash: Child protection under fire*. Thousand Oaks, CA: Sage.

Finkelhor, D. (2009). The prevention of childhood sexual abuse. *The Future of Children, 19*(2), 169–194.

Finkelhor, D., Ji, K., Mikton, C., & Dunne, M. (2013). Explaining lower rates of sexual abuse in China. *Child Abuse & Neglect, 37*, 852–860.

Fisher, A. K., Mackey, T. D., Langendoen, C., & Barnard, M. (2016). Child and interviewer race in forensic interviews. *Journal of Child Sexual Abuse, 25*(7), 777–792.

Flam, A. M., & Haugstvedt, E. (2013). Test balloons? Small signs of big events: A qualitative study on circumstances facilitating adults' awareness of children's first signs of sexual abuse. *Child Abuse & Neglect, 37*, 633–642.

Fontes, L. A., & Plummer, C. A. (2010). Cultural issues in disclosures of child sexual abuse. *Journal of Child Sexual Abuse, 19*, 491–518.

Giardino, A. P., Desai, K., Lew, D., Doerr, M. J., & Nojadera, B. (2016). Child sexual abuse prevention: Are safe environment training programs effective? A topical review of the literatures. *Jacobs Journal of Pediatrics, 3*(1), 006.

Goodman-Brown, T. B., Edelstein, R. S., Goodman, G. S., Jones, D. P. H., & Gordon, D. S. (2003). Why children tell: A model of children's disclosure of sexual abuse. *Child Abuse & Neglect, 27*, 525–540.

Hamilton, G., Brubacher, S. P., & Powell, M. B. (2016). Expressions of shame in investigative interviews with Australian aboriginal children. *Child Abuse & Neglect, 51*, 64–71. https://doi.org/10.1016/j.chiabu.2015.11.004.

Hassan, M., Hotz, R., Killion, C., & Vicken, T. (2015). Young victims telling their stories of sexual assault in the emergency department. *Iss Ment Hlth Nurs, 36*, 944–952.

Hechler, D. (1988). *The battle and the backlash: The child sexual abuse war*. Lexington, MA: Lexington Books.

Heger, A., Ticson, L., Velasquez, O., & Bernier, R. (2002). Children referred for possible sexual abuse: Medical findings in 2384 children. *Child Abuse & Neglect, 26*, 645–659.

Henry, N., & Powell, A. (2016). Technology-facilitated sexual violence: A literature review of empirical research. *Trauma, Violence, & Abuse, 19*(2). https://doi.org/10.1177/1524838016650189.

Hershkowitz, I., Horowitz, D., & Lamb, M. E. (2005). Trends in children's disclosure of abuse in Israel: A national study. *Child Abuse & Neglect, 29*, 1203–1214.

Hershkowitz, I., Lamb, M. E., Orbach, Y., Katz, C., & Horowitz, D. (2012). The development of communicative and narrative skills among preschoolers: Lessons from forensic interviews about child abuse. *Child Development, 82*(2), 611–622.

Hershkowitz, I., Lanes, O., & Lamb, M. E. (2007). Exploring the disclosure of child sexual abuse with alleged victims and their parents. *Child Abuse & Neglect, 31*, 111–123.

Hudson, K. M., & Giardino, A. P. (1996). Child abuse and neglect. In L. A. Kurtz, P. W. Dowrick, S. E. Levy, & M. L. Batshaw (Eds.), *Handbook of developmental disabilities: Resources for interdisciplinary care* (pp. 542–553). Gathersburg, MD: Aspen.

Hunter, S. V. (2011). Disclosure of child sexual abuse as a life-long process: Implications for health professionals. *The Australian and New Zealand Journal of Family Therapy, 32*, 159–172.

Individuals with Disabilities Education Act (IDEA). (1990). Pub. L. No. 101–476.

Jackson, S., Newall, E., & Backett-Milburn, K. (2015). Children's narratives of sexual abuse. *Child and Family Social Work, 20*, 322–332.

Jensen, K. J., Gulbrandsen, W., Mossige, S., Reichelt, S., & Thersland, O. A. (2005). Reporting possible sexual abuse: A qualitative study on children's perspectives and the context for disclosure. *Child Abuse & Neglect, 29*, 1395–1413.

Jobe-Shields, L., Swiecicki, C. C., Fritz, D. R., Stinnette, J. S., & Hanson, R. (2016). Post traumatic stress and depression in non-offending caregivers of sexually abused children: Association with parenting practices. *J Child Sex Ab, 25*(1), 110–125.

Jones, L., Mitchell, K., & Finkelhor, D. (2012). Trends in youth internet victimization: Findings from three youth internet safety surveys 2000-2010. *Journal of Adolescent Health, 50*, 179–186.

Kellogg, N., & The Committee on Child Abuse and Neglect. (2005). The evaluation of sexual abuse in children. *Pediatrics, 116*, 506–512.

Kempe, C. H. (1978). Sexual abuse, another hidden pediatric problem: The 1977 C. Anderson Aldrich Lecture. *Pediatrics, 62*, 382–289.

Kogan, S. M. (2004). Disclosing unwanted sexual experiences: Results from a national sample of adolescent women. *Child Abuse & Neglect, 28*, 147–165.

Lainpelto, K., Isaksson, J., & Lindblad, F. (2016). Does information about neuropsychiatric diagnoses influence evaluation of child sexual abuse allegations? *Journal of Child Sexual Abuse, 25*(3), 276–292. https://doi.org/10.1080/10538712.2016.1145164.

Leach, C., Powell, M. B., Sharman, S. J., & Anglim, J. (2017). The relationship between children's age and disclosures of sexual abuse during forensic interviews. *Child Maltreatment, 22*(1), 79–88.

Leclerc, B., & Wortley, R. (2015). Predictors of victim disclosure in child sexual abuse: Additional evidence from a sample of incarcerated adult sex offenders. *Child Abuse & Neglect, 43*, 104–111.

Lippert, T., Cross, T. P., Jones, L., & Walsh, W. (2009). Telling interviewers about sexual abuse: Predictors of child disclosure at forensic interviews. *Child Maltreatment, 14*, 100–113.

London, K., Bruck, M., Ceci, S. J., & Shuman, D. W. (2005). Disclosure of child sexual abuse: What does the research tell us about ways that children tell? *Psychology, Public Policy and Law, 11*, 194–226.

London, K., Bruck, M., Wright, D. B., & Ceci, S. J. (2008). Review of the contemporary literature on how children report sexual abuse to others: Findings, methodological issues, and implications for forensic interviewers. *Memory, 16*, 29–47.

Madden, M., Lenhart, A., Cortesi, S, & Gasser, U (2013). Teens and mobile apps privacy. Pew Research Center. Retrieved from http://www.pewinternet.org/2013/08/22/teens-and-mobile-apps-privacy/

Malloy, L. C., Brubacher, S. P., & Lamb, M. E. (2011). Expected consequences of disclosure revealed in investigative interviews with suspected victims of child sexual abuse. *Applied Developmental Science, 15*(1), 8–19.

Malloy, L. C., Lyon, T. D., & Quas, J. A. (2007). Filial dependency and recantation of child sexual abuse. *Journal of the American Academy of Child & Adolescent Psychiatry, 46*, 162–170.

Malloy, L. C., Mugno, A. P., Rivard, J. R., Lyon, T. D., & Quas, J. A. (2016). Familial influences on recantation in substantiated child sexual abuse cases. *Child Maltreatment, 21*(3), 256–261.

Mansbridge, J., & Shames, S. (2008). Toward a theory of backlash: Dynamic resistance and the central role of power. *Politics & Gender Journal, 4*(4), 623–634.

Masilo, G. M., & Davhana-Maselesele, M. (2016). Experiences of mothers of sexually abused children in north-west province, post disclosure. *Curationis, 39*(1), a1659. https://doi.org/10.4102/curationis.v39i1.1659.

McElvaney, R., Greene, S., & Hogan, D. (2012). Containing the secret of child sexual abuse. *Journal of Interpersonal Violence, 27*, 1155–1175.

Melville, J. D., Kellogg, N. D., Perez, N., & Lukefahr, J. L. (2014). Assessment for self-blame and trauma symptoms during the medical evaluation of suspected sexual abuse. *Child Abuse & Neglect, 38*, 851–857.

Merriam-Webster. (n.d.) Backlash. In Merriam-Webster.com dictionary. Retrieved from https://www.merriam-webster.com/dictionary/backlash

Mian, M., Wehrspan, W., Klajner-Diamond, H., LeBaron, D., & Winder, C. (1986). Review of 125 children 6 years of age and under who were sexually abused. *Child Abuse & Neglect, 10*, 223–229.

Mitchell, K. J., Finkelhor, D., Jones, L., & Wolak, J. (2010). Use of social networking sites in online sex crimes against minors: An examination of national incidence and means of utilization. *Journal of Adolescent Health, 47*, 183–190.

Mitchell, K., Finkelhor, D., & Wolak, J. (2007). Youth internet users at risk for the Most serious online sexual solicitations. *American Journal of Preventive Medicine, 32*(6), 532–537.

Mitchell, K., Jones, L. M., Finkelhor, D., & Wolak, J. (2011). Internet-facilitated commercial sexual exploitation of children: Findings from a nationally representative sample of law enforcement agencies in the United States. *Sexual Abuse: A Journal of Research and Treatment, 23*(1), 43–71.

Myers, J. (Ed.). (1994). *The backlash: Child protection under fire.* Thousand Oaks, CA: SAGE.

NPR. (2012). *Penn State abuse scandal: A guide and timeline.* Retrieved from https://www.npr.org/2011/11/08/142111804/penn-state-abuse-scandal-a-guide-and-timeline

Orbach, Y., & Lamb, M. E. (2007). Young children's references to temporal attributes of allegedly experienced events in the course of forensic interview. *Child Development, 78*, 1100–1120.

Pew Research Center. (2017). *Social media fact sheet.* Retrieved January 12, 2017, from http://www.pewinternet.org/fact-sheet/social-media/

Pintello, D., & Zuravin, S. (2001). Intrafamilial child sexual abuse: Predictors of postdisclosure maternal belief and protective action. *Child Maltreatment, 6*, 344–352.

Rakovec-Felser, Z., & Vidovic, L. (2016). Maternal perceptions of and responses to child sexual abuse. *Zdrav Var, 55*(2), 124–130.

Reitsema, A. M., & Grietens, H. (2016). Is anybody listening? The literature on the dialogical process of child sexual abuse disclosure reviewed. *Trauma, Violence, & Abuse, 7*(3), 330–340.

Saul, J., & Audage, N. C. (2007). *Preventing child sexual abuse within youth-serving organizations: Getting started on policies and procedures. Centers for Disease Control and Prevention.* Atlanta, GA: National Center for Injury Prevention and Control.

Schaeffer, P., Leventhal, J. M., & Gottsegen Asnes, A. (2011). Children's disclosures of sexual abuse: Learning from direct inquiry. *Child Abuse & Neglect, 35*, 343–352.

Sedlak, A. J., Mettenburg, J., Basena, M., Petta, I., McPherson, K., Greene, A., & Li, S. (2010). *Fourth National Incidence Study of child abuse and neglect (NIS–4): Report to congress, executive summary.* Washington, DC: U.S. Department of Health and Human Services, Administration for Children and Families.

Shattuck, A., Finkelhor, D., Turner, H., & Hamby, S. (2016). Children exposed to abuse in youth-serving organizations: Results from national sample surveys. *JAMA Pediatrics, 170*(2), e154493.

Sjöberg, R. L., & Lindblad, F. (2002). Limited disclosure of sexual abuse in children whose experiences were documented by videotape. *The American Journal of Psychiatry, 159*, 312–314.

Statista Research Department. (2019). Number of social network users in the United States as of January 2015, by age. Retrieved from http://www.statista.com/statistics/243582/us-social-media-ser-age-groups/

Steward, M. S., Bussey, K., Goodman, G. S., & Saywitz, K. J. (1993). Implications of developmental research for interviewing children. *Child Abuse & Neglect, 17*, 25–37.

Sullivan, P. M., & Knutson, J. F. (2000). Maltreatment and disabilities: A population-based epidemiological study. *Child Abuse and Neglect, 24*(10), 1257–1274.

Tashjian, S. M., Goldfarb, D., Goodman, G. S., Quas, J. A., & Edelstein, R. (2016). Delay in disclosure of non-parental child sexual abuse in context of emotional and physical maltreatment: A pilot study. *Child Abuse & Neglect, 58*, 149–159.

The Boston Globe. (2002). Scores of priests involved in sex abuse cases. Retrieved from https://www.bostonglobe.com/news/special-reports/2002/01/31/scores-priests-involved-sex-abuse-cases/kmRm7JtqBdEZ8UF0ucR16L/story.html

Topping, K. J., & Barron, I. G. (2009). School-based child abuse prevention programs: A review of effectiveness. *Review of Educational Research, 79*(1), 431–463.

Turchi, R. M., & Giardino, A. P. (2019). Medical home and health care systems. In M. L. Batshaw, N. J. Roizen, & L. Pellegrino (Eds.), *Children with disabilities* (pp. 799–817). Baltimore, MD: Paul H. Brookes.

Turner, H. A., Vanderminden, J., Finkelhor, D., Hamby, S., & Shattuck, A. (2011). Disability and victimization in a national sample of children and youth. *Child Maltreatment, 16*, 275–286.

Ullman, S. E. (2007). Relationship to perpetrator, disclosure, social reactions, and PTSD symptoms in child sexual abuse survivors. *Journal of Child Sexual Abuse, 16*, 19–36.

U.S. Census Bureau. (2011). School-aged children with disabilities in U.S. metropolitan statistical areas: 2010. Retrieved from https://www.census.gov/library/publications/2011/acs/acsbr10-12.html

U.S. Department of Health and Human Services, Health Resources and Services Administration, Maternal and Child Health Bureau (USDHHS). (2014). *Child health USA 2014*. Rockville, MA: Department of Health and Human Services.

U.S. Department of Health and Human Services Health Resources & Services Administration, Maternal and Child Health Bureau (USDHHS). (2019). Children with Special Health Care Needs. Retrieved from https://mchb.hrsa.gov/maternal-child-health-topics/children-and-youth-special-health-needs

van Toledo, A., & Seymour, F. (2016). Caregiver needs following disclosure of child sexual abuse. *Journal of Child Sexual Abuse, 25*(4), 403–414. https://doi.org/10.1080/10538712.2016.1156206.

Wang, L.-H., Lu, T., & Tsai, C.-H. (2016). Children's disclosure of sexual abuse during early forensic psychiatric evaluation in southern Taiwan. *Journal of the Formosan Medical Association, 115*, 1–7. https://doi.org/10.1016/j.jfma.2016.05.002.

Weatherred, J. L. (2015). Child sexual abuse and the media: A literature review. *Journal of Child Sexual Abuse, 24*(1), 16–34. https://doi.org/10.1080/10538712.2015.976302.

Wolak, J., & Finkelhor, D. (2013). Are crimes by online predators different from crimes by sex offenders who know youth in-person? *Journal of Adolescent Health, 53*, 736–741.

Wolak, J., Finkelhor, D., & Kimberly, M. (2008). Online "predators" and their victims: Myths, realities, and implications for prevention treatment. *American Psychology, 63*, 111–128.

Wolak, J., Finkelhor, D., & Mitchell, K. (2009). *Trends in arrests of "online predators"*. Durham, NH: Crimes Against Children Research Center.

Ybarra, M., & Mitchell, K. (2008). How risky are social networking sites? A comparison of places online where youth sexual solicitation and harassment occurs. *Pediatrics, 121*, e350–e357.

Chapter 4
Compassion Fatigue, Burnout, and Coping Strategies among Child-Serving Professionals

4.1 Ending Violence against Children

According to a 2016 World Health Organization (WHO) report, half of all children aged 2–17 years (up to 1 billion children) in 96 countries are exposed to one or more forms of interpersonal violence every year (WHO, 2016). Childhood exposure to violence has a dose–response relationship to adult causes of morbidity and mortality, including mental illness and suicide attempts, alcoholism, substance abuse, sexually transmitted infections, and chronic health problems such as heart disease, stroke, and lung disease. (Centers for Disease Control and Prevention, 2018). The WHO has detailed seven evidence-based strategies for ending violence against children (WHO, 2016):

- Implementation and enforcement of laws.
- Challenging restrictive norms and values.
- Creating safe environments.
- Providing parent and caregiver support.
- Strengthening incomes and economic development.
- Creating response and support services.
- Teaching education and life skills.

A large cadre of resilient, long-serving social workers, mental health clinicians, law enforcement officials, prosecutors, educators, victim advocates, nurses, and physicians is needed to implement and sustain these seven WHO strategies and potentially prevent short- and long-term consequences of childhood interpersonal violence. To be effective and long-serving, each professional must adopt individualized, positive coping mechanisms, ideally within a workplace culture that supports and values self-care and resilience.

© The Author(s) 2020
T. S. Hinds, A. P. Giardino, *Child Sexual Abuse*, SpringerBriefs in Public Health, https://doi.org/10.1007/978-3-030-52549-1_4

4.2   Compassionate Service and Idealism

Compassion is often the impetus to serve maltreated children and can be a source of strength for child-serving professionals. Not all child-serving professionals will be affected in the same manner following exposure to maltreated children, and not all child-serving professionals develop negative trauma symptomatology. However, for many child-serving professionals, dispensing daily doses of compassion can have adverse side effects. Secondary trauma and burnout are often cited as critical reasons that significant numbers of child-serving professionals leave their professions or reduce hours at work. In one study, nearly 40% of former multidisciplinary team members cited job stress and perceived burnout as significant factors in their decision to leave their teams (Bennett, 2005).

Multiple individual and structural factors contribute to job stress. For instance, child-serving professionals working with maltreated children and their families may hold assumptions or expectations that are overly idealistic or unrealistic:

- Family problems are always manageable and we have the tools to be helpful.
- I know *exactly* what my role is in relation to families and children I serve.
- Parents and children want my help and will view my efforts positively.
- Because of my role as a helper, I will be safe (e.g., I should be able to tolerate client verbal abuse and visiting unsafe neighborhoods).
- I will not do harm.
- As a mental health practitioner, I should always be empathic with any client.
- I am engaged in activities that are valued by others.
- I will always receive the support of my colleagues.
- I approach my work with a clear idea of my biases and have ways to keep them out of my judgments and reactions (Azar, 2000).

Violation of these assumptions and expectations may have adverse effects on child-serving professionals, including secondary stress, compassion fatigue, and burnout.

4.3   Secondary Traumatic Stress, Compassion Fatigue, and Burnout

Compassion fatigue refers to the physical and psychological stress suffered by the professional that results from exposure to the traumatized individual (Figley, 1995, 2012). Characteristics of compassion fatigue include reduced capacity for empathy, desensitization to client or patient experiences, a decrease in quality of care, and an increase in clinical errors (Figley, 1995, 2012). Compassion fatigue can adversely affect direct service to children and relationships with colleagues and family members. It may result in post-traumatic stress disorder (PTSD), anxiety, and/or depression (Figley, 1995, 2012). In a study conducted by Conrad and Kellar-Guenther, approximately 50% of child protection caseworkers and their supervisors reported experiencing high or extremely high levels of compassion fatigue (Conrad & Kellar-Guenther, 2006). It appears that responding to children's trauma, as opposed to adult trauma, may further increase the professional's risk of compassion fatigue (Figley, 1995, 2012).

Burnout occurs in an environment of continued physical and psychological stress and generally consists of three components: emotional exhaustion, depersonalization, and a reduced sense of personal accomplishment (Conrad & Kellar-Guenther, 2006). Effects can also include fatigue, physical complaints, anxiety, and/or depression (Figley, 1995, 2012). Burnout contributes to compassion fatigue and is associated with an erosion of idealism (Figley, 1995, 2012). Nearly 8% of social workers or their supervisors report their risk of burnout to be high or extremely high (Conrad & Kellar-Guenther, 2006). Although the majority of research involves social workers and mental health professionals, any member of a child-serving multidisciplinary team is at risk for compassion fatigue and burnout. Attorneys who have long hours of direct contact with clients have higher rates of burnout, depression, and post-traumatic stress symptoms compared with their administrative colleagues (Levin et al., 2011). In this study of attorneys, gender, age, years of service, size of local office, and personal history of trauma did not predict these adverse symptoms (Levin et al., 2011). The law enforcement literature does hint at the possibility of gender differences in compassion fatigue and burnout. Among male detectives investigating sex crimes against children, open communication with a spouse/life-partner was associated with a lower risk of burnout (Lane, Lating, Lowry, & Martino, 2010). This is consistent with other studies that highlight the importance of a personal support system. In contrast, among female detectives, open communication was not associated with lower risk of compassion fatigue and burnout (Lane et al., 2010). Female detectives also reported less quality time with their partners and less sexual wellness than male detectives (Lane et al., 2010). Researchers speculated these findings may be related to female detectives' awareness that an open communication style with a male spouse/life-partner may be potentially detrimental if that style seeps into their investigative work with predominantly male perpetrators of child sex crimes (Lane et al., 2010).

4.4 Positive Coping Strategies

Resilient child-serving professionals are critical if there is to be increased prevention, recognition, and treatment of the global problem of child maltreatment. Therefore, researchers have attempted to understand how child-serving professionals with career longevity mitigate or prevent compassion fatigue and burnout. Among social workers and their supervisors, coping strategies influence the incidence of burnout (Anderson, 2000). **Frontline "veteran" social workers with at least two years of experience are more likely to report the use of active coping strategies (problem-solving, cognitive restructuring) compared with problem**

avoidance, withdrawal, and self-criticism as a way to manage job stress (Anderson, 2000). Avoidant strategies appear to correlate with increased emotional exhaustion, one of the three components of burnout. While two-thirds of veteran social workers report emotional exhaustion, their use of problem-solving and cognitive restructuring appear to ameliorate depersonalization and a reduced sense of personal accomplishment, the second and third components of burnout (Anderson, 2000). **Cognitive restructuring involves less focus on idealistic or unrealistic assumptions and increased focus on more flexible assumptions about individuals** (Azar, 2000):

- Individuals (parents/supervisees/supervisors/colleagues) do the best they can.
- Individuals need to feel a sense of mastery in their role.
- Individuals have difficulty being easy on themselves.
- Seeking help is dangerous.
- Individuals are ambivalent about wanting help.
- Individuals expect you to tell them "you're doing a bad job".
- There is no one right way for individuals to work.
- Change can feel dangerous to the person who has to do something differently.
- Change is slow to occur.

Several common coping strategies also emerge from studies of homicide and sex crime investigators, including investigators who view pornographic images (Johnson, 2009; Miller, 2009):

- Focus on gathering information and maintaining intellectual curiosity about details of the crime and offender's pathology.
- Creation of a physical workspace where explicit and/or confidential content is not in plain sight.
- Maintenance of a professional attitude and manner of speech.
- Engagement with peers as a form of support and expert consultation.
- Compartmentalization of family and work life.
- Recognition that healthy humor is needed to cope with cynicism, rage, disgust, and occupational stressors.

In both the child welfare and law enforcement literature, humor is noted to be both a positive coping strategy and a sign of distress. Studies have been done about the associations among secondary traumatic stress, self-deprecating humor, humor about society/human behavior, humor at the expense of victims, humor at the expense of offenders, and humor containing sexual innuendo (Craun & Bourke, 2015). Healthy humor (lighthearted and/or self-deprecating humor) lowers secondary stress and encourages bonding among team members with shared experiences. Unhealthy humor belittles victims or other professionals (Craun & Bourke, 2015; Miller, 2009). Unhealthy humor, such as humor at the expense of the child victim and humor about physically threatening or emotionally disturbing situations is a warning sign of poor coping and indicates a need for intervention(s) to target secondary traumatic stress (Craun & Bourke, 2015; Miller, 2009). Among investigators of sex crimes against children, the frequency with which humor is used at the expense of the victims is related to high secondary traumatic stress scores (Craun & Bourke, 2015). There also appears to be a relationship among joking about human behavior, greater distrust of the world, and high secondary traumatic stress scores (Craun & Bourke, 2015). Humor containing sexual innuendo is viewed as socially undesirable. However, there does not appear to be a statistically significant relationship between the use of humor at the expense of offenders and humor containing sexual innuendo and secondary traumatic stress (Craun & Bourke, 2015).

Similar to community-based child-serving professionals, multidisciplinary hospital-based child-serving professionals also report high levels of burnout and job stress (Bennett, 2005). Child abuse pediatricians experience conflicted relationships with families, adversarial courtroom experiences, lawsuits against the professional, and financial pressures because of multiple hours of uncompensated work (Flaherty, Schwartz, Jones, & Sege, 2013). Child abuse pediatricians who have practiced an average of 16 years have experienced threats to their personal safety (52%), complaints to supervisors (50%) and licensing bodies (13%), negative stories in the media (23%), and malpractice suits (16%) (Flaherty et al., 2013). A frequently cited positive coping strategy by child abuse pediatricians involves the development of support networks, not only within hospital teams, but also across systems and with colleagues at other institutions (Flaherty et al., 2013). **Support networks and relationships are used to discuss cases, process emotions, maintain perspective, and reduce feelings of isolation** (Flaherty et al., 2013). Not surprisingly, the effectiveness of child protection teams increases in an atmosphere of collegiality, social support from colleagues, and interdisciplinary collaboration and feedback (Kistin, Tien, Bauchner, Parker, & Leventhal, 2010). Child abuse pediatricians have described multiple coping strategies to maintain resilience (Flaherty et al., 2013):

- Development of personal and professional support networks.
- Limit setting at work and clear boundaries between home and work life.
- Use of all vacation days.
- Extracurricular activities that do not involve violence.

Based on themes that emerge from the social services, law enforcement, and medical literature on compassion fatigue and burnout, child-serving professionals will likely benefit from increased use of positive coping strategies, appropriate balance between their professional and personal lives, and increased use of co-worker and supervisory support systems. Formal psychological and psychiatric treatment should also be considered on an individual basis. Typically, child maltreatment investigations involve months of information gathering and multiple interviews of children, non-offending caregivers, collateral witnesses, and suspects. Law enforcement literature reminds child-serving professionals that positive coping strategies must be deployed immediately among first responders and also redeployed on a regular basis throughout the course of investigations (Miller, 2009).

4.5   Organizational Support

Ideally, individual efforts are complemented by organizational strategies to support child-serving professionals, their supervisors, and administrative support staff. Organizational strategies that foster resilience and prevent and address secondary traumatic stress include regular, ongoing organizational interventions (National Child Traumatic Stress Network, 2018):

- Clinical supervision.
- Reflective supervision.
- Trauma case load balance.
- Workplace self-care groups.
- Flextime scheduling.
- Enhancements to employee safety.
- Secondary trauma trainings for clinical and administrative staff and organizational leaders.
- Trainings of organizational leaders on the continuous assessment of secondary trauma.
- External partnerships with secondary trauma intervention providers.

Some organizations have the resources to regularly host professional resilience trainings, such as the US-based Accelerated Recovery Program (ARP) for Compassion Fatigue developed by Gentry, Baranowsky, and Dunning (2002), that have been proven to reduce secondary trauma symptoms and compassion fatigue. Organizations also utilize freely available validated tools such as the Professional Quality of Life Scale (ProQOL) and the Vicarious Trauma Toolkit (VTT). The ProQOL is a free self-administered screening tool that evaluates compassion satisfaction, burnout, and compassion fatigue (ProQOL Measure, 2019). It has been in use since 1995 and is currently available in 25 languages. ProQOL helps individuals determine how to maximize personal resilience. It can also be used during organizational planning to maximize an organizational culture of wellness. The Vicarious Trauma Toolkit (VTT) assesses organizational readiness and describes processes and resources to achieve a work environment that promotes compassion, personal and professional growth, and self-care (U.S. Department of Justice, n.d.). Organizational strategies that lessen the impact of secondary stress, compassion fatigue and burnout are described in the VTT based on discipline—Victim Services, Emergency Medical Services, Fire Services, and Law Enforcement (U.S. Department of Justice, n.d.). Child welfare-focused organizations can also utilize the Secondary Traumatic Stress Informed Organization Assessment (STSI-OA) Tool to determine the extent to which their organizations are able to respond to secondary traumatic stress (National Child Traumatic Stress Network, 2014). The most trauma-informed organizations develop and sustain formal and informal strategies which move beyond debriefings after critical incidents and difficult cases to also address daily occupational related stressors and barriers to employee resilience and professional fulfillment.

4.6 Summary

Each child-serving professional has the ability to positively impact the life of a child. Each professional will also be personally and professionally affected during their service, sometimes in a potentially detrimental manner. Thus, the most emotionally healthy child-serving professionals and trauma-informed organizations will be those who utilize positive strategies that mitigate the effects of secondary traumatic stress and lessen the risk of burnout and compassion fatigue. Individual and organizational efforts to develop a culture of wellness must be nurtured if the seven WHO strategies to end violence against children are to be broadly and effectively implemented and sustained.

References

Anderson, D. (2000). Coping strategies and burnout among veteran child protection workers. *Child Abuse & Neglect, 24*(6), 839–848. https://doi.org/10.1016/s0145-2134(00)00143-5.

Azar, S. (2000). Preventing burnout in professionals and paraprofessionals who work with child abuse and neglect cases: A cognitive behavioral approach to supervision. *Journal of Clinical Psychology, 56*(5), 643–663. https://doi.org/10.1002/(sici)1097-4679(200005)56:5<643::aid-jclp6>3.0.co;2-u.

Bennett, S. (2005). Burnout, psychological morbidity, job satisfaction, and stress: A survey of Canadian hospital based child protection professionals. *Archives of Disease in Childhood, 90*(11), 1112–1116. https://doi.org/10.1136/adc.2003.048462.

Conrad, D., & Kellar-Guenther, Y. (2006). Compassion fatigue, burnout, and compassion satisfaction among Colorado child protection workers. *Child Abuse & Neglect, 30*(10), 1071–1080. https://doi.org/10.1016/j.chiabu.2006.03.009.

Craun, S., & Bourke, M. (2015). Is laughing at the expense of victims and offenders a red flag? Humor and secondary traumatic stress. *Journal of Child Sexual Abuse, 24*(5), 592–602. https://doi.org/10.1080/10538712.2015.1042187.

Figley, C. (1995). *Compassion fatigue*. New York, NY: Brunner/Mazel.

Figley, C. (Ed.) (2012). Compassion fatigue. In *Encyclopedia of trauma: An interdisciplinary guide*. New York, NY: SAGE. doi:https://doi.org/10.4135/9781452218595.

Flaherty, E., Schwartz, K., Jones, R., & Sege, R. (2013). Child abuse physicians: Coping with challenges. *Evaluation & the Health Professions, 36*(2), 163–173. https://doi.org/10.1177/0163278712459196.

Gentry, J., Baranowsky, A., & Dunning, K. (2002). The accelerated recovery program (ARP) for compassion fatigue. In C. Figley (Ed.), *Treating compassion fatigue* (pp. 123–137). New York, NY: Brunner-Routledge.

Johnson, S. (2009). Impact of pornography on forensic mental health and law enforcement professionals: Effective coping strategies. *International Journal of Emergency Mental Health, 11*(2), 93–96.

Kistin, C., Tien, I., Bauchner, H., Parker, V., & Leventhal, J. (2010). Factors that influence the effectiveness of child protection teams. *Pediatrics, 126*(1), 94–100. https://doi.org/10.1542/peds.2009-3446.

Lane, E., Lating, J., Lowry, J., & Martino, T. (2010). Differences in compassion fatigue, symptoms of posttraumatic stress disorder and relationship satisfaction, including sexual desire and functioning, between male and female detectives who investigate sexual offenses against children: A pilot study. *International Journal of Emergency Mental Health, 12*(4), 257–266.

Levin, A., Albert, L., Besser, A., Smith, D., Zelenski, A., Rosenkranz, S., & Neria, Y. (2011). Secondary traumatic stress in attorneys and their administrative support staff working with trauma-exposed clients. *The Journal of Nervous and Mental Disease, 199*(12), 946–955. https://doi.org/10.1097/nmd.0b013e3182392c26.

Miller, L. (2009). Criminal investigator stress: Symptoms, syndromes, and practical coping strategies. *International Journal of Emergency Mental Health, 11*(2), 87–92.

National Child Traumatic Stress Network. (2014) Secondary traumatic stress Informed Organization Assessment (STSI-OA) Tool.. Retrieved from https://www.nctsn.org/resources/secondary-traumatic-stress-informed-organization-assessment-stsi-oa-tool.

National Child Traumatic Stress Network. (2018). Organizational secondary traumatic stress [Webinar]. Retrieved from https://www.nctsn.org/resources/organizational-secondary-traumatic-stress.

ProQOL Measure. (2019). Retrieved from https://proqol.org/ProQol_Test.html.

U.S. Department of Justice, Office of Justice Programs, Office for Victims of Crime. (n.d.). Vicarious Trauma Toolkit. https://vtt.ovc.ojp.gov/about-the-toolkit

World Health Organization (WHO). (2016). INSPIRE: Seven strategies for ending violence against children. Retrieved from http://www.who.int/violence_injury_prevention/violence/inspire/en/

Chapter 5
Policy Direction: Focus on Prevention

5.1 Introduction

Child sexual abuse (CSA) is a significant public health threat to children affecting at least 58,114 to more than 135,500 on an annual basis (USDHHS, 2019; Sedlak, Mettenburg, Winglee, Ciarico, & Basena, 2010), as discussed in the opening chapter of this monograph. (See Chap. 1 for more detailed discussion). Averting our gaze from the problem of CSA is just not a responsible approach to a threat to the health and well-being of children and adolescents. The healthcare response to CSA is hinged on understanding the risk and being able to recognize a case where CSA might be a diagnostic possibility. Next, the healthcare professional is typically called upon to use their skills to conduct a thorough evaluation (see Chap. 2 for a description). And, finally, when there is a concern for possible CSA, the healthcare professional must comply with their mandated responsibility of reporting the case to child protection and law enforcement authorities for investigation. This response, however, occurs after the abuse has occurred. Instead, healthcare providers along with many in child advocacy and among the public want to see effective prevention efforts so that the abuse can be avoided before the child is harmed. Since C. Henry Kempe (1978) first referred to CSA as another hidden pediatric epidemic (Kempe, 1978), a great deal of effort has been invested in CSA prevention efforts, but numerous studies and meta-analyses have been uniformly disappointing in demonstrating that these CSA prevention efforts have in fact reduced the incidence or prevalence of actual sexual victimization of children in our society. While the epidemiologic data supports a trend of decreasing incidence of substantiated cases of CSA, the discussion in Chap. 1 raises concerns about viewing the reduction of substantiated claims as the same as an actual reduction in victimization. Prior to claiming that victory for children, better methods will be required to base that finding on solid scientific inquiry.

This chapter will explore general prevention concepts as they apply to CSA and then will discuss two different but complementary approaches to CSA prevention,

© The Author(s) 2020
T. S. Hinds, A. P. Giardino, *Child Sexual Abuse*, SpringerBriefs in Public Health, https://doi.org/10.1007/978-3-030-52549-1_5

namely child-focused education that empowers children to protect themselves and adult-focused training that assists parents and other caregivers to supervise and monitor the children's environment in a way that creates as safe an environment as possible. The chapter concludes with an appendix of a list of organizations that promote CSA prevention, many of which provide excellent resources via regularly updated, publicly available websites.

5.2 Background

5.2.1 CSA Prevention vs. Child Physical Abuse Prevention

In a companion monograph on child physical abuse, the authors provided a detailed description of the public health model for child abuse prevention (Hinds & Giardino, 2017). In short, efforts designed to prevent a health problem can be categorized based on the targeted population and are designated as primary, secondary, or tertiary prevention types (Hinds & Giardino, 2017). Primary prevention targets the general population at all levels of risk and employs universal intervention techniques offered to everyone. Secondary prevention targets an at-risk population and uses targeted intervention techniques to identify and provide services and supports to those at risk. Finally, tertiary prevention is akin to treatment and targets those already affected and aims to stop new incidents by treating those who have already experienced the problem or issue. This public health approach has been widely adopted for the prevention of child physical abuse. However, CSA is a different clinical and social phenomenon than is child physical abuse (and child neglect) and etiologies and issues surrounding risk for sexual victimization are not the same as for child physical abuse. As such, the prevention approaches will likely need to be different as well. For example, Daro highlights these differences along the lines of the public health prevention model (Daro, 1994). First, she describes the prevention approach for physical abuse as spanning all of the prevention strategies:

> Historically, the prevention of physical abuse and neglect has developed on all three levels. The most common primary prevention strategies include respite care, crisis hot lines, home visitor programs, parenting education classes, and support groups. Political efforts to improve the social service safety net and to combat the environmental hazards children face also are viewed as vital components in a comprehensive child abuse prevention effort. Secondary prevention strategies include educational and support services for parents facing significant challenges based upon their current situation (for example, teen parenthood, economic stress, violent household, presence of substance abuse, social isolation) or childhood history (for example, abuse as a child). Tertiary prevention efforts include therapeutic or supportive interventions targeted to those who have abused or neglected their children. (Daro, 1994)

Next, Daro explicitly contrasts this physical abuse prevention approach to that seen with child sexual abuse prevention:

The prevention of child sexual abuse has followed a different developmental path in two critical respects--the targeting of the potential victim rather than the potential perpetrator and an emphasis on primary rather than secondary or tertiary prevention. Unlike the efforts to alter adult behavior in cases of physical abuse or neglect, the prevention of child sexual abuse has largely focused on altering the behavior of children, through group-based instruction for children on how to protect themselves from or respond to sexual assault or abuse. In many instances, this education is provided through elementary and secondary schools, although several national youth organizations have developed their own curricula ... While these programs do include information for parents and teachers, their primary focus is on strengthening the potential victim's capacity to resist assault. (Daro, 1994).

By far and away, the majority of CSA prevention programs are school-based or youth serving organization-based safe environment training programs that seek to raise awareness among the children about the problem of CSA, their risk, and appropriate ways to disclose if they are subjected to CSA. Evaluations of these programs will be described in fuller detail below. Much of current CSA prevention practice hinges on educating the children themselves so that they can be empowered to protect themselves. While these child-focused education programs are relatively widespread, they are coming under thoughtful scrutiny (Rudolph & Zimmer-Gembeck, 2018; Del Campo & Fávero, 2019). As a result, a growing movement is emerging that advocates for a stronger adult focus whereby parents and adults in caregiving roles are trained in the knowledge and skills necessary to create a safe environment and on how best to supervise and monitor that environment to keep children as safe as possible from the risk and occurrence of CSA. Martyniuk and Dworkin, writing for the National Sexual Violence Resource Center, summarize this growing awareness about the complementary value of weaving together both child- and adult-focused CSA prevention efforts:

Traditional child sexual abuse prevention programs are of value because they provide information, support and empowerment. However, concerns have been raised that these programs target children and inappropriately place the burden of prevention on the child. Indeed, child sexual abuse occurs as a result of many factors working together, all of which are beyond the control of the child. Additionally, critics suggest that it may be unrealistic to expect a child to assert power over someone whom they may trust and who is in a position of authority, older and likely stronger than them. ... In the end, it is the responsibility of individuals to not violate children in any way and for communities to actively engage in the prevention of child sexual abuse and safeguard the well-being of children. (Martyniuk & Dworkin, 2011b)

5.2.2 Calls for CSA Prevention

The Center for Disease Control and Prevention (CDC) is at the forefront of the public health effort to prevent all forms of child maltreatment, including child physical abuse, child neglect, and CSA. The CDC, through the National Center for Injury Prevention and Control's Division of Violence Prevention, issued a broad outline of how the nation can address child maltreatment prevention entitled Essentials for Childhood: Creating Safe, Stable, Nurturing Relationships, and Environments

(CDC, 2019a). This positive, forward thinking, capacity building document, while not specifically addressing the details of CSA prevention, does provide an overarching framework for national policy and guidance around a stepwise approach to creating the type of safe, stable, nurturing environment free from harm within which most would want children to grow and develop. Table 5.1 summarizes the four goals and their related action steps contained in the CDC's Essentials document:

About 15 years prior to the appearance of the CDC's Essentials document, the Children's Hospital and Health Center San Diego (now Rady Children's

Table 5.1 CDC approach to child well-being and child maltreatment prevention

Essentials for childhood: steps to create safe, stable, nurturing relationships, and environments	
Term	**Definition**
Safety	The extent to which a child is free from fear and secure from physical or psychological harm within their social and physical environment.
Stability	The degree of predictability and consistency in a child's social, emotional, and physical environment.
Nurturing	The extent to which children's physical, emotional, and developmental needs are sensitively and consistently met.
Goals	**Steps**
Raise awareness and commitment to promote safe, stable, nurturing relationships, and environments	• Partner with others to build commitment. • Develop a shared agenda (vision, goals, and metrics). • Consistent and strategic messaging.
Use data to inform solutions	• Use partnerships to help identify, gather, and synthesize relevant data. • Take stock of what data already exist in your community. • Identify and fill critical data gaps. • Use the data to support other action goals and steps.
Create the context for healthy children and families through norms change and programs	• Promote the community norm that we all share responsibility for the well-being of children. • Promote positive community norms about parenting programs and acceptable parenting behaviors. • Implement evidence-based programs for parents and caregivers.
Create the context for healthy children and families through policies	• Identify and assess which policies may positively impact the lives of children and families in your community. • Provide decision-makers with information on the benefits of evidence-based strategies and rigorous evaluation.

Adapted from "Essentials for Childhood: Creating Safe, Stable, Nurturing Relationships and Environments" by the Centers for Disease Control and Prevention, National Center for Injury Prevention and Control, Division of Violence Protection, 2019, https://www.cdc.gov/violenceprevention/childabuseandneglect/essentials.html

Hospital-San Diego) hosted an invitational conference of national experts to explore the possibility and potential value of a call to action around child maltreatment prevention. According to Blair Sadler, CEO of the children's hospital at the time,

> We are well aware of the fact that several extensive studies and commissions, including the US Advisory Board on Child Abuse and Neglect, have examined the state of child abuse and neglect in America and have completed excellent reports. Unfortunately, according to many of the individuals who participated in these efforts, they have not served as an effective catalyst to galvanize a nationally coordinated action agenda. (Sadler, 1999, p. 956)

While this National Call to Action may not have galvanized a large as desired outcome, a number of white papers emanated from this conference that provided those focused on prevention with valuable perspectives. Among the most useful was provided by Dr. David Chadwick, the emeritus director for child abuse services at the hosting children's hospital. Dr. Chadwick talks about the time and persistence that those who seek to foster social change must be prepared for. He refers to these social change agents as "keepers." In Chadwick's words:

> We also should remember that all-important social change is effected by sets of determined persons who can sustain efforts over long periods of time. In the case of child abuse, we may need another century. To be effective, we require keepers of a plan who will devote many decades of their lives to the effort. The keepers will keep the message alive. It will take sweat and tears. These keepers must recruit successors with similar dedication. Who, among you, are the keepers? Who will be willing to step forward and work tirelessly to keep the message alive? (Chadwick, 1999)

Among the "keepers" of the vision for a world free of CSA are those on the National Coalition to Prevent Child Sexual Exploitation. The Prevention Coalition identified six areas, or Six Pillars of Prevention, in which policies can have the most impact (National Coalition to Prevent Child Sexual Exploitation, 2015):

Six Pillars of Prevention
1. Strengthen Youth Serving Organizations' sexual abuse and exploitation prevention capacity.
2. Support the healthy development of children.
3. Promote healthy relationships and sexuality education for children and youth.
4. End the demand for children as sexual commodities.
5. Have sustainable funds for prevention.
6. Prevent initial perpetration of child sexual abuse and exploitation.

This material was reprinted, with permission, from the National Coalition to Prevent Child Sexual Abuse and Exploitation's Six Pillars for Prevention.

Building on this work is the Committee for Children, a global nonprofit dedicated to research-based educational programs that promote social-emotional skills and which prevent bullying and CSA. The Committee for Children issued six policy recommendations related to CSA prevention:

- Develop a broad, national, evidence-informed educational program to identify the signs of child sexual abuse and take steps to prevent it. Support research, targeted cultural messages, and outreach efforts (to populations most at risk) to start a national conversation on eliminating child sexual abuse and promoting child safety.
- Develop a national technical assistance center that, at a minimum, provides states with information on evidence-based prevention programs, funds evaluation of promising practices, runs a national hotline for individuals affected by child sexual abuse, advocates for more uniform definitions of child sexual abuse and guidelines for child sexual abuse reporting, and is the repository of training programs for mandatory reporters.
- Incorporate a two-generational approach in all child sexual abuse prevention work that targets the child and the child's parents/caregivers.
- Develop culturally specific educational programs and reporting tools that would enable cultural communities at risk to more readily recognize and report abuse and seek help.
- Advocate for funding to support both evidence-based prevention strategies and research to evaluate promising prevention practices.
- End statute of limitation laws for reporting child sexual abuse. (Committee for Children, 2016).

Another group of "keepers" in the effort to rid children of the risk and trauma related to CSA are those with the national advocacy organization Prevent Child Abuse America. In their policy statement aimed at eliminating the threat of CSA, Prevent Child Abuse America harkens to the collective responsibility to prevent CSA, spanning support for social services systems to promoting awareness training and rigorous research on that training to ensure its needed impact. Table 5.2 describes Prevent Child Abuse America's six-point advocacy effort aimed at prevention CSA.

5.2.3 Research and Evaluation on Existing CSA Prevention Programs

Clearly, a call to action to prevent CSA requires actual programs that operationalize the public health concepts into practical, concrete action steps. To date, the Committee for Children identifies two types of CSA prevention efforts, (1) education and training focused on adults in the children's environment, and (2) programming focused on skills training in children (2016). These two types of programs

Table 5.2 Prevent child abuse America's CSA Prevention approach

Action	Description
Raising awareness of the unacceptability of child sexual abuse and promoting the notion that stopping child sexual abuse is everyone's responsibility	A powerful public education message must be transmitted to the general public, encouraging society to recognize that child sexual abuse is everyone's problem and responsibility. The goal of such public education efforts is to eliminate any tolerance for sexual abuse or confusion over what society condones as appropriate interactions between adults and children.
Educating the public, especially policymakers, about the true nature of child sexual abuse	The wide dissemination of accurate information to the public, especially to policymakers, will help break the silence and taboo that surrounds child sexual abuse, and may facilitate the formulation of effective solutions to the problem.
Rigorously evaluating and strengthening existing child sexual abuse prevention programs	Current child abuse prevention programs are focused primarily on educating preschool and elementary school children on how to recognize instances of abuse and teaching them personal safety skills. Research yields little evidence that such programs actually prevent the occurrence of child abuse. Although program evaluations demonstrate short-term knowledge gain, they fail to establish a link between such knowledge gain and the prevention of child sexual abuse. ... Demonstrating effectiveness is a challenging task, mainly because of the methodological shortcomings of existing evaluations.
Shifting the prevention of child sexual abuse from children to adults	Adults must exercise an affirmative obligation to safeguard children from sexual abuse ... While strengthening existing child sexual abuse prevention programs, efforts must be made to create programs that shift the responsibility of child sexual abuse prevention from children to adults and public institutions ... Additional efforts are needed, including parent education in methods for reducing the risk of child sexual abuse and training for professionals and other caregivers who work with children to recognize and appropriately respond to sexually reactive behavior.
Exploring, evaluating, and strengthening new approaches to preventing child sexual abuse	New, cutting-edge approaches are being developed to prevent child sexual abuse. Such approaches complement the criminal justice and child protective systems, but focus more on accountability, rehabilitation, and restitution than on punishment ... Such approaches, including fostering survivor leadership, circles of accountability and support, targeted public messages directed at perpetrators and would-be perpetrators of child sexual abuse, and child sexual offender treatment, should be further explored, rigorously evaluated, and strengthened.
Making mental health services available to all those affected by child sexual abuse	Children who have been sexually abused may face severe and long-term psychological consequences. Mental health services, especially if timely, can help ease some of these consequences ... Mental health services to those engaging in abusive behavior can help them address stressors that often lead to sexual abuse, helping end such abuse.

Adapted from "Preventing Child Sexual Abuse Position Statement" by Prevent Child Abuse America, 2016, http://preventchildabuse.org/wp-content/uploads/2016/02/6a-Position-Paper-on-Preventing-CSA.pdf

incorporate the six pillars of prevention discussed above in a practical manner. With regard to CSA prevention, most programs to some degree or another also incorporate the early conceptualization put forth by Finkelhor known as the four preconditions of for CSA: (1) motivation of the perpetrator, (2) overcoming internal inhibitions, (3) overcoming external inhibitions, and (4) overcoming child resistance (Finkelhor, 1984). CSA prevention efforts most frequently focus on preconditions (3) and (4), namely ensuring adequate barriers to abuse in the child's environment and empowering children in appropriate ways to resist and not keep secrets. Over the past three decades, a significant effort has been made to evaluate CSA prevention efforts, concentrated mostly on child-focused skills training occurring in the school setting. Table 5.3 provides a brief description of several of these evaluation efforts.

With the recent focus over the past decade on adult-focused education or training for parents and other adults who work with children, one can expect that an equally robust effort to evaluate the adult-focused programs will be comparable to the child-focused studies listed in Table 5.3.

5.2.3.1   Child-Focused Skills Training

CSA prevention programs using child-focused skills training tend to include information on what CSA is, ownership over one's body and who can touch what parts, self-protection skills, the need to avoid self-blame if one is abused, and the disclosure process to alert of potential or actual CSA (Giardino, Desai, Lew, Doerr, & Nojadera, 2016). Despite this general content, programs tend to vary in terms of format, type of and training for instructors, and the frequency over which the training is provided (Daro, 1994). Wurtele provides a relatively recent critique of the child-focused personal safety educational programs designed to prevent CSA (Wurtele, 2009). On the positive side, the child-focused CSA programs do appear to provide children with the opportunity to learn about CSA concepts and, depending on the teaching method, to also learn personal safety skills as well as to avoid blaming themselves if abuse occurs (Wurtele, 2009). According to a summary by Martyniuk and Dworkin, researchers have consistently found a number of benefits to CSA prevention programs:

- Increased knowledge about child sexual abuse.
- Increased self-protective knowledge and skills, and increased use of these self-protective skills.
- Earlier disclosure of abuse, which could prevent further abuse from occurring and allow the child to be treated for the abuse.
- Shorter duration of abuse.
- Increased positive feelings about self and decreased negative feelings about self (Martyniuk & Dworkin, 2011b).

Knowledge gains from prevention programs usually last for several months and may last as long as a year (Topping & Barron, 2009). Because of this, it is important

Table 5.3 Scholarly evaluation of CSA Prevention efforts

Citation	Summary	Comments
Reppucci, N. D., & Haugaard, J. J. (1989). Prevention of child sexual abuse: Myth or reality. American Psychologist, 44(10), 1266–1275.	A review of the content and effects of selected child sexual abuse prevention programs and the underlying assumptions driving the programs.	One of the earliest studies looking at an aggregate of prevention programs.
Madak, P. R. & berg, D. H. (1992). The prevention of sexual abuse: An evaluation of "talking about touching." Canadian Journal of Counseling, 26(1), 29–40.	An evaluation of "talking about touching" in five elementary schools in Canada.	Detailed evaluation of one specific program; measured student knowledge, surveyed teachers who delivered the program, and surveyed parents.
Daro, D.A. (1994). Prevention of child sexual abuse. The future of children: Sexual Abuse of children, 4 (2). Center for the Future of children. The David and Lucille Packard Foundation.	A review of 17 well-designed studies of child sexual abuse prevention programs.	Overview of child sexual abuse prevention underlying principles along with the thoughtful topical review.
Rispens, J., Aleman A., & Goudena, P. P. (1997). Prevention of child sexual abuse victimization: A meta-analysis of school programs. Child Abuse & Neglect, 21(10), 975–987.	A meta-analysis used to calculate results of 16 evaluation studies of school-based child sexual abuse prevention programs.	Comprehensive review of the existing studies to date to gain a big-picture overview of the effectiveness of prevention programs.
Plummer, C. A. (2001). Prevention of child sexual abuse: A survey of 87 programs. Violence and Victims, 16(5), 575–588.	A survey of 87 child sexual abuse prevention programs, with an emphasis on how they function in their community contexts.	Broad look at implementation challenges and realities of prevention programs.
Bolen, R. M. (2003). Child sexual abuse: Prevention or promotion? Social Work, 48(2), 174–185.	A review of school-based child sexual abuse prevention programs and a comparison of such programs to a healthy relationship paradigm.	Largely a theoretical discussion of the underlying assumptions, methods, and goals of child-focused versus male-focused prevention programs.
Finkelhor, D. (2009). The prevention of childhood sexual abuse. The Future of Children, 19(2), 169–194.	An examination of initiatives to prevent child sexual abuse, including law enforcement initiatives, school-based educational programs, and counseling programs.	Evidence-based evaluation of most prevalent programs and policies aimed at preventing child sexual abuse by a leading scholar in the field.

(continued)

Table 5.3 (continued)

Citation	Summary	Comments
Mikton, C. & Butchart, A. (2009). Child maltreatment prevention: a systematic review of reviews. Bulletin of the World Health Organization, 87(5), 353–361.	An examination of 26 reviews of child sexual abuse prevention programs from a global public health perspective.	Global public health evaluation of variety of child abuse prevention programs, including home visits, parent education programs, media campaigns, and child-focused sexual abuse prevention training.
Topping, K. J. & Barron, I. G. (2009). School-based child abuse prevention programs: a review of effectiveness. Review of Educational Research, 79(1), 431–463.	Review of 22 studies of the effectiveness of school-based child sexual abuse prevention programs.	Comprehensive review of the current data on the effectiveness of prevention programs.
Wurtele, S.K. (2009) preventing sexual abuse of children in the twenty-first century: Preparing for challenges and opportunities. Journal of Child Sexual Abuse 18(1):1–18.	Description of scope and consequences of child sexual abuse and a critique of child-focused personal safety education programs.	Thoughtful description of conceptual underpinnings of child sexual abuse prevention educational efforts. The critique uses arguments based on the existing evidence to challenge assumptions that are driving the field.
Lalor, K. & McElvaney, R. (2010). Child sexual abuse, links to later sexual exploitation/high-risk sexual behavior, and prevention/ treatment programs. Trauma, Violence and Abuse, 11(4), 159–177.	Examination of the nature and incidence of child sexual abuse, the long-term effects of such abuse on children, and review of the literature on prevention strategies and effective interventions.	Thorough overview on the nature, incidence and effects of child sexual abuse, as well as various prevention efforts, including media campaigns, school-based programs, therapy of abusers, and therapy of children and their families.
Rudolph, J., Zimmer-Gembeck, M.J., Shanley, D.C., Hawkins, R. (2018). Child sexual abuse prevention opportunities: Parenting, programs, and the reduction of risk. Child Maltreatment 23(1):96-106.	Exploration of the conceptual underpinnings of shifting towards adult-focused child sexual abuse prevention efforts.	A detailed walk-through of the literature that supports the argument for adult-focused training, especially of parents as an important child sexual abuse prevention effort.
Del Campo, A. & Fávero, M. (2019) effectiveness of programs for the prevention of child sexual abuse: a comprehensive review of evaluation studies. European Psychologist 25:1–15.	A review of 70 child sexual abuse prevention studies published between 1981 and 2017	Comprehensive review of a significant body of literature.

to reinforce the skill and knowledge gains through continued prevention efforts throughout childhood. Indeed, additional program sessions have been found to help children maintain and increase their knowledge and skills about child sexual abuse prevention (Topping & Barron, 2009).

On the negative side, however, some have raised concerns that children may experience anxiety, may be more likely to misinterpret nurturing touches and potentially make false accusations of CSA (Wurtele, 2009), but research has shown little evidence of these negative effects. While some children report that the program made them feel worried or scared, no significant increase in anxiety among program participants has been found, and few teachers or parents reported behavior problems or emotional distress (Wurtele, 2009). Likewise, few program participants have been found to misinterpret nurturing touches or make false allegations (Wurtele, 2009). Another topical review addresses the potential negative effects of child-focused CSA prevention programs by offering:

> Scholarly research has found limited evidence of any negative effects caused by child-focused sexual abuse prevention programming .... While some studies found an increase in worry in children following training, this may actually be an appropriate reaction, in that it demonstrates that children are taking the threat of sexual abuse seriously ... Only a small number of children reported any other negative reaction, such as loss of sleep or appetite, nightmares, bedwetting, or behavioral issues ... Most of the negative effects reported by children are small, mild, and brief in duration ... (Giardino et al., 2016)

A uniform criticism of the research on child-focused CSA programs is the inability to document that these programs directly decrease the incidence or prevalence of CSA. The sad reality is that Finkelhor's observation still rings true today, namely "No strong scientific evidence points as yet in the direction of one strategy or program to prevent sexual abuse" (Finkelhor, 2009). With that said, Finkelhor reiterates the positives regarding the child-focused CSA prevention skills training:

- School-based CSA prevention programs are among the most evaluated prevention strategies to date and the results are "encouraging".
- School-based prevention efforts in other domains such as the prevention of bullying and delinquency have been shown to be effective which lends support to CSA prevention.
- School-based CSA preventions appear to be a non-stigmatizing and efficient communication vehicle for the prevention message.
- School-based CSA prevention programs have the added benefit of providing: (1) a deterrent message to potential perpetrators who are aware of the children's education in this area of risk, and (2) an encouraging message to bystanders for the need to intervene to protect a child from abuse.
- Owing to the near universal access to all children, school-based programs are an efficient way to target nearly all children for a prevention message (2009).

5.2.3.2 Adult-Focused Education and Training

With the above discussion of child-focused CSA programming in mind, there are increasing efforts to shift the focus of CSA prevention efforts to the adults in the child's environment. The CDC recommends additional research on CSA with the overarching goal of informing effective prevention efforts to stop the abuse before it occurs:

> Adults must take the steps needed to prevent child sexual abuse. Adults are responsible for ensuring that all children have safe, stable, nurturing relationships and environments. Resources for child sexual abuse have mostly focused on treatment for victims and criminal justice-oriented approaches for perpetrators. While these efforts are important after child sexual abuse has occurred, little investment has been made in primary prevention, or preventing child sexual abuse BEFORE it occurs. Thus, limited effective evidence-based strategies for proactively protecting children from child sexual abuse are available. More resources are needed to develop, evaluate, and implement evidence-based child sexual abuse primary prevention strategies to ensure that all children have safe, stable, nurturing relationships and environments. (CDC, 2019b)

With the goal of shifting CSA efforts towards educating and training the adults in the children's environment, Martyniuk and Dworkin (2011a) describe a five-goal plan for training parents. See Table 5.4 for a description.

Rudolph and colleagues also argue for the inclusion of parents in the prevention effort. Specifically, they highlight that parents can play a significant role as

Table 5.4 CSA prevention training goals for parents

Goal	Description
Teach parents how to educate their children about sexual abuse prevention	• Discuss topics without scaring child. • Teach child how to protect him/herself. • Teach child how to tell what is and isn't abuse. • Tailor concepts to child's skills and developmental levels.
Teach parents how to protect their children from child sexual abuse	• Understand that most people who sexually abuse children are known to the victim and the victim's family. • Know the characteristics of people who sexually abuse children and the ways they manipulate parents and children.
Teach parents to recognize signs that abuse is occurring and take steps to stop it	• Identify signs of abuse. • Respond appropriately to disclosures. • Monitor sexual development. • Learn about local child abuse reporting systems and services for victims and families.
Teach parents how to strengthen healthy family dynamics	• Strengthen parent–child relationships. • Encourage supportive and open communication. • Discourage secrecy.
Support prevention efforts directed at children and other adults	• Reinforce prevention messages in multiple contexts. • Discuss prevention concepts in natural settings.

This material was adapted, with permission, from the National Sexual Violence Resource Center's publication entitled Child Sexual Abuse Prevention: Programs for Adults. This guide is available by visiting www.nsvrc.org

protectors of their children directly by erecting strong external barriers via supervision, monitoring, and involvement, and indirectly by encouraging their children's sense of self-efficacy, well-being, and self-esteem (Rudolph & Zimmer-Gembeck, 2018). Little research exists around the adult-focused CSA prevention efforts, but emerging evidence suggests that parents view having a close relationship with the child and supervising and monitoring social settings as important (Rudolph, Zimmer-Gembeck, Shanley, & Hawkins, 2018). Interestingly, the majority of studies suggest that discussion of sexual abuse prevention at home is not seen by parents as necessarily an essential element to CSA prevention (Rudolph et al., 2018).

Broadening the discussion to adults other than the parents who work with children may be promising. Martyniuk and Dworkin point out the few studies in this area show that such training leads to a positive impact on the adults' knowledge of CSA, better understanding of the mandated reporting responsibility they may have, and adults being better equipped to make a decision about the need to report (Martyniuk & Dworkin, 2011a). Additionally, they describe two goals for the non-parental adult CSA prevention training listed in Table 5.5.

In the years to come, additional research will be necessary to determine how effective the adult-focused CSA prevention efforts are for both parents and other adults who work with children. While a call for shifting the burden of CSA prevention away from the children towards the adults is conceptually sound, there is need for scientifically rigorous research and evaluation to confirm this shift is having the needed protective effect.

Table 5.5 CSA prevention training goals for adults who work with children

Goal	Description
Teach people who work with children how to educate children about child sexual abuse prevention	• Review the topics to be presented to children. • Teach presentation skills.
Teach people who work with children how to identify and report child sexual abuse	• Discuss physical and behavioral signs of abuse. • Review the local reporting system. • Discuss what to do with suspicions of abuse. • Review services for victims and families. • Role-play interventions and reactions to disclosures.

This material was adapted, with permission, from the National Sexual Violence Resource Center's publication entitled Child Sexual Abuse Prevention: Programs for Adults. This guide is available by visiting www.nsvrc.org

5.3   Conclusion

Clearly, the above discussion demonstrates a great deal of collective professional work that has been done to prevent CSA, and, at the same time, suggests just how much work is likely to be needed to achieve the goal of safe, stable, and nurturing environments for children free from CSA. Much of this future work will rely on carefully done research, which should guide the investment of time and resources in

Table 5.6 Gaps in research and practice for CSA Prevention

Domain/Gap	Action steps
Improve surveillance systems and data collection	• Develop and implement surveillance systems to assess child sexual abuse perpetration and victimization in real-time to measure recent and lifetime exposure. • Use standard definitions and measures of child sexual abuse to increase availability and quality of data. • Collect data focused on victimization and perpetration of all forms of child sexual abuse to improve our understanding of all aspects of child sexual abuse.
Strengthen and develop evidence-based policies, programs, and practices	• Further evaluate evidence-based approaches in different populations, communities, and settings. • Identify, develop, and evaluate programs and practices that reduce youth and adult perpetrated CSA. • Develop and evaluate comprehensive primary prevention programs, practices, and policies that address individual, relationship, community, and societal factors that impact child sexual abuse.
Increase understanding of risk and protective factors	• Develop research that assesses exposure to child sexual abuse and risk and protective factors over time to inform primary prevention efforts. • Identify risk and protective factors for child sexual abuse at multiple levels of influence—Individual, relationship, community, and societal. • Examine and identify distinctions between different types of child sexual abuse perpetration to inform primary prevention efforts. • Determine how risk and protective factors for child sexual abuse perpetration interact with other forms of violence perpetration to better prevent all forms of violence.
Disseminate and implement evidence-based policies, programs, and practices	• Act on the best available evidence now—Scale-up, implement, and communicate information about existing evidence-based strategies to prevent child sexual abuse. • Explore how to adapt the existing evidence-based interventions for different populations and settings. • Identify strategies for effectively communicating best practices for child sexual abuse prevention among practitioners, researchers, clinicians, and others working directly with children.

Adapted from "Preventing Child Sexual Abuse" by the Centers for Disease Control and Prevention, National Center for Injury Prevention and Control, Division of Violence Protection, 2019, www.cdc.gov/violenceprevention/childabuseandneglect/childsexualabuse.html

such an important prevention effort directed towards the elimination of CSA. The CDC identified the research gaps in CSA prevention from their public health perspective, which include attention to surveillance and data collection systems, development of evidence-based policies and practice, increased understanding of risk and protective factors, and finally, better dissemination and implementation of evidence-based programs, policies, and practices. Table 5.6 provides a more detailed set of action steps within each of these domains.

Rudolph and Zimmer-Gembeck, in their critique of current CSA programming, offer a set of perspectives on where policy, practice, and research regarding CSA prevention ought to move:

- The lack of evidence that child-focused programs help children to avoid abuse requires more efforts to rigorously evaluate the widespread use of these programs.
- CSA prevention and protection information and skills training for parents should become part of all parenting programs.
- Those working with vulnerable families should be aware of the risk factors of CSA and work with parents to better protect their children.
- Future research needs to move beyond parental discussion of CSA with their children as the focal point of CSA prevention to the role of parenting behaviors such as communication, monitoring, and involvement.
- Further research should evaluate the effect on protective parenting behaviors of parenting programs with a CSA component. (Rudolph & Zimmer-Gembeck, 2018).

Thus, much has been done regarding CSA prevention, and much still needs to be done. Harkening back to Blair Sadler's vision for the National Call to Action to end all forms of maltreatment, including CSA, "Let us begin ..." (Sadler, 1999).

Appendix: Organizations that Promote CSA Prevention

Organization	Website description
Child Welfare Information Gateway http://www.childwelfare.gov	Child Welfare Information Gateway promotes the safety, permanency, and well-being of children, youth, and families by connecting child welfare, adoption, and related professionals as well as the public to information, resources, and tools covering topics on child welfare, child abuse and neglect, out-of-home care, adoption, and more. A service of the Children's Bureau, Administration for Children and Families, U.S. Department of Health and Human Services, we provide access to print and electronic publications, websites, databases, and online learning tools for improving child welfare practice, including resources that can be shared with families.

Organization	Website description
Child Welfare League of America http://www.cwla.org	Child Welfare League of America (CWLA) leads and engages its network of public and private agencies and partners to advance policies, best practices, and collaborative strategies that result in better outcomes for children, youth, and families that are vulnerable. CWLA's focus is children and youth who may have experienced abuse, neglect, family disruption, or a range of other factors that jeopardize their safety, permanence, or well-being. CWLA also focuses on the families, caregivers, and the communities that care for and support these children.
Darkness to Light http://www.darkness2light.org	Darkness to Light empowers adults to prevent, recognize, and react responsibly to child sexual abuse through awareness, education, and stigma reduction … trainings are the only evidence-informed, adult-focused child sexual abuse prevention trainings proven to increase knowledge and change behavior. Through the combination of research, education, and community advocacy, darkness to light uses a social behavior change approach to pioneer new training initiatives that bring child sexual abuse to the attention of the broader cultural conversation. Over the years, nearly two million adults in 76 countries have been trained to protect children through the efforts of more than 12,000 certified instructors and authorized facilitators.
National Center for Missing & Exploited Children http://www.missingkids.com	The National Center for Missing & Exploited Children (NCMEC) is a private, nonprofit 501(c)(3) corporation whose mission is to help find missing children, reduce child sexual exploitation, and prevent child victimization. NCMEC works with families, victims, private industry, law enforcement, and the public to assist with preventing child abductions, recovering missing children, and providing services to deter and combat child sexual exploitation.
National Children's Advocacy Center http://www.nationalcac.org	The National Children's Advocacy Center (NCAC), located in Huntsville, Alabama, revolutionized the United States' response to child sexual abuse. Since its creation in 1985, the NCAC has served as a model for the 1000+ children's advocacy centers now operating in the United States and in more than 34 countries throughout the world, with 9 more currently in development. The CAC model of a multidisciplinary team approach, developed through the vision of former congressman Cramer and a group of key individuals, pulled together law enforcement, criminal justice, child protective services, and medical and mental health workers onto one coordinated team.

Organization	Website description
National Sexual Violence Resource Center http://www.nsvrc.org	The National Sexual Violence Resource Center (NSVRC) is the leading nonprofit in providing information and tools to prevent and respond to sexual violence. NSVRC translates research and trends into best practices that help individuals, communities, and service providers achieve real and lasting change. NSVRC also works with the media to promote informed reporting. Every April, NSVRC leads Sexual Assault Awareness Month, a campaign to educate and engage the public in addressing this widespread issue.
Prevent Child Abuse America http://www.preventchildabuse.org	Prevent Child Abuse America (PCAA) is the nation's oldest and largest nonprofit organization dedicated to the primary prevention of child abuse and neglect. Through a national chapter network and evidence-based programs—Including the signature healthy families America home visiting model—PCAA helps prevent abuse and neglect before it can begin. PCAA works to help to strengthen families, support communities, and foster safe, stable, and nurturing relationships that help children thrive.
Stop It Now! http://www.stopitnow.org	Stop It Now! was founded by Fran Henry, a survivor of childhood sexual abuse who learned firsthand that standard approaches to keeping children safe from child sexual abuse at that time did not respond to the complex relationships surrounding most abuse. In 2015, Stop It Now! became an affiliate of Klingberg Family Centers, a private, nonprofit multi-service agency based in New Britain, CT. Stop It Now! prevents the sexual abuse of children by mobilizing adults, families, and communities to take actions that protect children before they are harmed.
Stop the Silence http://www.stopcsa.org	Stop the Silence began in 2002 as a coalition of multi-ethnic and state groups that came together to comprehensively address child sexual abuse. Pamela Pine, PhD, MPH, an international health and development specialist, launched programming to address the pandemic and the critical need for a comprehensive response for this very complex issue. Dr. Pine organized Stop the Silence into a nonprofit organization in 2004 given the need for a structure from which to provide adequate, essential, and comprehensive programming. Activities include research, media advocacy, training, community outreach and education, policy development, and support for direct services.

References

Centers for Disease Control and Prevention, National Center for Injury Prevention and Control, Division of Violence Protection (CDC). (2019a). Essentials for childhood: Creating safe, stable, nurturing relationships and environments. Retrieved from https://www.cdc.gov/violenceprevention/childabuseandneglect/essentials.html

Centers for Disease Control and Prevention, National Center for Injury Prevention and Control, Division of Violence Protection (CDC). (2019b). Preventing child sexual abuse. www.cdc.gov/violenceprevention/childabuseandneglect/childsexualabuse.html

Chadwick, D. (1999). The message. *Child Abuse & Neglect, 23*(10), 957–961. https://doi.org/10.1016/S0145-2134(99)00072-1.

Committee for Children. (2016). Prevention of child sexual abuse: A policy briefing. Retrieved from https://www.cfchildren.org/wp-content/uploads/policy-advocacy/Committee-for-Children_Policy-White-Paper_Protecting-Our-Children-from-Sexual-Abuse_FA18.pdf

Daro, D. A. (1994). Prevention of child sexual abuse. *The Future of Children, 4*(2), 198–223. https://doi.org/10.2307/1602531.

Del Campo, A., & Fávero, M. (2019). Effectiveness of programs for the prevention of child sexual abuse: A comprehensive review of evaluation studies. *European Psychologist, 25*, 1–15. https://doi.org/10.1027/1016-9040/a000379.

Finkelhor, D. (1984). *Child sexual abuse: New theory and research.* NY: Free Press.

Finkelhor, D. (2009). The prevention of childhood sexual abuse. *The Future of Children, 19*(2), 169–194. https://doi.org/10.1353/foc.0.0035.

Giardino, A. P., Desai, K., Lew, D., Doerr, M. J., & Nojadera, B. (2016). Child sexual abuse prevention: Are safe environment training programs effective? A topical review of the literatures. *Jacobs Journal of Pediatrics, 3*(1), 006.

Hinds, T. S., & Giardino, A. P. (2017). *Child physical abuse: Current evidence, clinical practice, and policy directions.* Cham, Switzerland: Springer Nature.

Kempe, C. H. (1978). Sexual abuse, another hidden pediatric problem: The 1977 C. *Anderson Aldrich Lecture. Pediatrics, 62*, 382–289.

Martyniuk, H. & Dworkin, E. (2011a). Child sexual abuse prevention: Programs for adults.. National Sexual Violence Resource Center. Retrieved from https://www.nsvrc.org/sites/default/files/2012-03/Publications_NSVRC_Guide_Child-Sexual-Abuse-Prevention-programs-for-adults.pdf

Martyniuk, H. & Dworkin, E. (2011b). Child sexual abuse prevention: Programs for children National Sexual Violence Resource Center Retrieved from https://www.nsvrc.org/sites/default/files/Publications_NSVRC_Guide_Child-Sexual-Abuse-Prevention-programs-for-children.pdf

National Coalition to Prevent Child Sexual Abuse and Exploitation. (2015). Six pillars for prevention. Retrieved from www.preventtogether.org

Prevent Child Abuse America (2016). Preventing Child Sexual Abuse Position Statement.. Retrieved from http://preventchildabuse.org/wp-content/uploads/2016/02/6a-Position-Paper-on-Preventing-CSA.pdf

Rudolph, J., & Zimmer-Gembeck, M. J. (2018). Reviewing the focus: A summary and critique of child-focused sexual abuse prevention. *Trauma, Violence & Abuse, 19*(5), 543–554. https://doi.org/10.1177/1524838016675478.

Rudolph, J., Zimmer-Gembeck, M. J., Shanley, D. C., & Hawkins, R. (2018). Child sexual abuse prevention opportunities: Parenting, programs, and the reduction of risk. *Child Maltreatment, 23*(1), 96–106. https://doi.org/10.1177/1077559517729479.

Sadler, B. (1999). The vision. *Child Abuse & Neglect, 23*(10), 955–956. https://doi.org/10.1016/S0145-2134(99)00066-6.

Sedlak, Andrea J., Mettenburg, Jane., Winglee, Marianne, Ciarico, Janet., Basena, Monica. (2010) *Fourth national incidence study of child abuse and neglect (NIS-4): Report to congress.* Washington, DC: U.S. Department of Health and Human Services, Administration for Children and Families. Retrieved from http://www.acf.hhs.gov/sites/default/files/opre/nis4_report_congress_full_pdf_jan2010.pdf

Topping, K. J., & Barron, I. G. (2009). School-based child abuse prevention programs: A review of effectiveness. *Review of Educational Research, 79*(1), 431–463.

U.S. Department of Health & Human Services, Administration for Children and Families, Administration on Children, Youth and Families, Children's Bureau (USDHHS) (2019). Child Maltreatment 2017. Retrieved from https://www.acf.hhs.gov/cb/research-data-technology/statistics-research/child-maltreatment

Wurtele, S. K. (2009). Preventing sexual abuse of children in the twenty-first century: Preparing for challenges and opportunities. *Journal of Child Sexual Abuse, 18*(1), 1–18. https://doi.org/10.1080/10538710802584650.

Index

© The Author(s) 2020
T. S. Hinds, A. P. Giardino, *Child Sexual Abuse*, SpringerBriefs in Public
Health, https://doi.org/10.1007/978-3-030-52549-1

Printed in the United States
By Bookmasters